THE GLOBAL
CATASTROPHE
THAT IS EVIDENCE-BASED

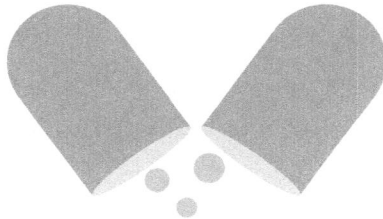

MEDICINE

How to Empower Doctors, Patients, Regulators
and Legislators to put Population Health
at the Centre of their Focus

CHRISTOPH
SCHNELLE PHD

ISBN 978-1-7638614-0-4 (Hardback)
ISBN 978-1-7638614-1-1 (Paperback)

Imprint: Christoph Schnelle

Interior Layout by Perseus Design

Note for the reader:
This book is intended for informational and educational purposes only. It does not constitute medical advice, diagnosis, or treatment. The content is not meant to be a substitute for professional medical advice, diagnosis, or treatment. Always seek the advice of a qualified healthcare provider with any questions you may have regarding a medical condition or treatment options. The author has made every effort to ensure the accuracy and completeness of the information contained in this book. However, the field of medicine is constantly evolving, and new research may supersede some of the information presented here. The author and publisher disclaim any liability, loss, or risk incurred as a consequence, directly or indirectly, of the use and application of any of the contents of this book. The discussion of vaccines and evidence-based medicine in this book is based on scientific literature and expert consensus available at the time of writing. However, medical knowledge and best practices may change over time. Readers should not rely solely on the information in this book to make healthcare decisions. This book may contain references to specific medical treatments, procedures, or products. These references do not imply endorsement or recommendation. Any decision regarding vaccination or medical treatment should be made in consultation with a qualified healthcare professional who can assess individual circumstances and medical history. The views and opinions expressed in this book are those of the author and do not necessarily reflect the official policy or position of any medical institution, organisation, or government agency. The author is not responsible for any adverse effects or consequences resulting from the use of any suggestions, preparations, or procedures described in this book. By reading this book, you acknowledge that you understand and agree to these terms and conditions.

CONTENTS

AUTHOR'S NOTE

A homage to doctors, medicine and research

Without medicine, humanity would be in a deep, dark hole as it was many times in the past millennia. Doctors and medicines have brought miracles of healing that have transformed our lives for the better, supported by research that has discovered many of those medicines and treatments.

This book is in support of true doctors, true medicine and true research, all of which support humanity to live healthier, longer and more productive lives.

To give an idea of the importance of medicine, consider the chaos that would ensue if for even one week no medical treatment could be given, and no medicine could be taken by anyone.

This greatness of purpose and execution have attracted a significant number of opportunists who are exploiting the goodwill for their own purposes in myriad ways. The exploitation and opportunism exist side-by-side with the true doctors, medicines and research and has increasingly taken over medicine with severe consequences for population health.

This book is about showing how that takeover has happened so individuals can make their own informed decisions and act from a much clearer understanding in relation to what is happening in medicine and therefore the world. The main mechanism used for this takeover has been what is referred to as evidence-based medicine. Evidence-based medicine in addition to its many benefits has been misused to corrupt research, to provide unsuitable medicines on a large scale and to neuter and intimidate doctors.

The election of Donald Trump and the elevation of Robert F. Kennedy Jr as of December, 2024 could provide the first strong move to reverse those trends of worsening population health.

Medicine had a pretty good run until the 1980s with a great deal of valuable new research findings and steadily increasing life expectancy. By the 1990s, the number of research findings had become unmanageably large in many areas of medicine and an existing medical research method, using the statistical methods provided by epidemiology, was combined with medical treatments by doctors of patients and rebranded as evidence-based medicine. This is when things started to go wrong as the book will reveal.

On a personal note, I studied for a Masters in Biostatistics in 2015 and had a conversation with a truly excellent teacher and professor about statistics. I stated what was obvious to me, that statistics is about truth. His reply was that statistics is not about truth but about probabilities. That floored me at the time and I missed the rejoinder that what are probabilities if not about truth?

I would like to take the opportunity to thank Professor Mark Jones, my thesis supervisor, a man of great integrity, a huge support and without whom the PhD would have taken years more to conclude. Truly a supervisor from Heaven.

Also, Nicola Lessing, my wife, editor, sounding board and source of wisdom. Oh, and joy, harmony, truth, love and stillness. There is an at-one-ness in our work and life and in the writing of this book.

CHAPTER 1

WHAT IS EVIDENCE-BASED MEDICINE?

One of the first definitions of evidence-based medicine was in the British Medical Journal (BMJ) written by David Sackett, medical doctor and researcher, in 1996 as this:

> *"The practice of evidence-based medicine means integrating individual clinical expertise with a critical appraisal of the best available external clinical evidence from systematic research."*(1)

The idea was that anybody who practises medicine can improve their practice by intelligently (critical appraisal) incorporating the best quality (systematic) medical research into their practice and therefore have access to much more knowledge as they do not need to only rely on their own clinical experience and knowledge.

For example, a single doctor, hospital, entire health district, country, the entire world, ideally would have access to the best available knowledge of the entire world when treating each patient and would therefore be much more capable than if they would solely rely on their own knowledge and experience.

There is a similarity to the current promise of Artificial Intelligence, giving everybody access to the world's knowledge in an easy-to-understand and easy-to-apply way. The next years will show how much of that promise will be kept, how reliable and helpful the knowledge, tools and work support that an artificial intelligence application provide are and what other consequences and potential misuse arise.

The same applies to evidence-based medicine. The quality and truthfulness of the "*best available external clinical evidence from systematic research*" is of critical importance in whether evidence-based medicine is a boon, a non-event, or in its overall application a crime or catastrophe. All apply at the moment. There are lifesaving and curing treatments, medicines that have no effect, there is declining population health such as the so far unstoppable rises in obesity, diabetes and other chronic illnesses plus the exponentially rising healthcare costs and there have been crimes against humanity.

A question to ask ourselves as population health continues to decline with various reasons given for that decline(2-8) whilst healthcare costs keep rising as a percentage of GDP,(9-14) is:

Is evidence-based medicine one of the reasons for the decline or is evidence-based medicine responsible for keeping an even bigger deterioration at bay?

Some might say that evidence-based medicine, in its much-documented support for individuals is a hero but add one consideration and everything looks very different:

> The way evidence-based medicine is practised today is that the process that decides what *"the best available clinical evidence"* is and has been thoroughly corrupted.

This book takes a comprehensive look at evidence-based medicine and its effect on doctors and patients, including many examples of the corruption and offers ways to respond to and apply evidence-based medicine in our current era.

The underlying weaknesses in today's application of evidence-based medicine are that truth has been substituted by rules and vested interests, that doctors have been disempowered and that patients are not held to their responsibilities.

Medicine is the art of healing people. If that is not the primary purpose of any medical activity, then that activity is at best interfering or may be actively harming people.

There are ways to deal with all of the weaknesses of medicine, whether one is an individual with no apparent power to change the way evidence-based medicine is applied or someone with any degree of power that can make changes to the application of any part of evidence-based medicine.

One of the most supportive acts in life to do what is necessary, is to know **what is actually going on** and I have regularly been quite shocked in the last nine years while researching for this book at what I found.

Being receptive and having one's eyes fully open while working at any capacity in or around healthcare or receiving healthcare is the first step to know what actions to take as an individual. For that it is critically important to have enough information and understanding for each individual to come to their own conclusions as to how to respond.

It was enormously enjoyable to put all this information together and to gain more and more understanding of the underlying causes and effects of the currently dominating paradigm of medicine that is evidence-based medicine.

In this book I will not shorten evidence-based medicine to EBM as using an acronym allows a false sense of detachment and diminishes the impact of both what is bad and what is good, what is beautiful and what is excellent of evidence-based medicine. I will not capitalise it either as evidence-based medicine is subordinate to the process of healing through medicine.

Some items are quite shocking and you may have reason to disagree with what follows but the writing is well supported by evidence.

Medicine has been around at least for millennia, with Imhotep in ancient Egypt(15) as *the first physician known by name in written history.*"(ibid.) but, medicine as used in the past, relied mostly on clinicians' experience and opinion. From the 1920s onwards, a number of well-working medical treatments were discovered, which by the 1980s led to an explosion in the number of medical research finding, so much so, that it made intuitive sense to make those many new research findings available to doctors in a systematic way by the 1990s. This was formalised under the umbrella term evidence-based medicine, which was a relabelling of the term 'epidemiology', allowing the concepts of epidemiology to be widely accepted under a different name.

So, what is evidence-based medicine *really* like?

Evidence-based medicine tells doctors what to do and is ubiquitously used in medicine. The 15 largest pharmaceutical companies alone spent $138 billion in 2022(16), a 43% increase from 2017, on medical research in addition to the spending by universities and governments that is the source of evidence-based medicine's authority.

I have put in many citations in order to provide evidence for what I write or to show where a reader can find more information. An example is that you can find historic details about evidence-based medicine in an article that I am referencing here:(17)

Should this vast spending on medical research mean we expect to live longer and have healthier lives on a population basis? Spending large amounts of money on sanitation certainly worked that way, increasing life expectancy substantially.(18, 19)

Since the rise of evidence-based medicine in 1996, life expectancy has not increased beyond the rate it was already increasing and it is now decreasing in countries like the United Kingdom and the United States.(20) We have much more chronic diseases and cancer even after adjusting for population age. The obesity epidemic is getting worse with people putting on weight faster the younger they are.(21)

The COVID-19 gestation and response exposed every negative aspect of evidence-based medicine, with this understanding moving from a derided conspiracy theory to an attacked conspiracy theory, to aspects of it being grudgingly accepted and it may well have become received and obvious knowledge by the time you read this.

We may be at stage one of the philosopher Arthur Schopenhauer's observation, translated by me from the original, slightly archaic German(22):

"... the fate which happened to every insight, especially the most important one, the truth, which was only a short victory celebration between the two long time spans in which she is being condemned as impossible and then belittled as trivial. Also the first of these fates tends to hit its originctor. – But life is short, and truth's effect reaches far and lives long: let us express the truth."

Which is commonly shortened to

"All truth passes through three stages. First, it is ridiculed. Second, it is violently opposed. Third, it is accepted as being self-evident."

A virus generated through medical research escapes or is released in the wild.(23-38) Even though the fatality rate is no higher in many countries than a bad flu(39) and successful early-stage remedies are found within months(40), we ended up with the following:

A vaccine campaign with 1.08 billion doses administered by mid-2024(41, 42) that may damage the immune system, perhaps seriously,(43-50) with emerging evidence of many deaths and injuries.(51, 52)

At the moment there are many sources considered credible or particularly credible that contradict or dispute any of the statements in the above paragraph, which is in line with Schopenhauer's statement about truth if those credible sources are incorrect, and at the moment there is no consensus about COVID-19's origin, fatality rate, treatment, or vaccination effectiveness.

In response to COVID-19, pandemic measures were taken such as lockdowns(53, 54) and masking mandates(55) that stifled development in many children(56, 57) and closed down a very large number of small businesses, all of which with the support of published medical research at the time.

Evidence-based medicine at best has no impact on longevity, nor does it prevent massive rises in chronic diseases. It is hugely expensive, can be used for research that has harming people as its purpose (gain-of-function research on pathogens)(58) or financial gain (research into foods that are hard to resist) and can be used and misused to enable deep damage to the population through 'treatments' that harm.(59-62)

One of the main reasons we have this state of affairs is that the gatekeepers to health, medical doctors, have been very effectively silenced or are complicit in allowing the above as it is genuinely dangerous for their livelihood if they speak up and there can be very substantial financial and career benefits in complying or being complicit.

The entire last two paragraphs are substantiated in this book.

Evidence-base medicine can point to many individual research findings that help in individual cases of sickness but its effect on population health has been at best negligible and is more likely harming and evidence-based medicine can be misused to very seriously harm population health.

A strong and authoritative medical profession would never allow the abuse that happened during COVID-19 and the ongoing takeover by evidence-based medicine through many useful but also many corrupt and often useless guidelines. Guidelines are useless for the many people who are multi-symptomatic and take multiple pharmaceuticals in response, as it is physically impossible to do research on more than a few interactions between multiple medicines. That means the research of evidence-based medicine has no answer for the majority of older people and the doctor is on their own.

So, what happened since evidence-based medicine rose in 1996? How have doctors been deauthorised and are now allowing such levels of abuse?

A substantial reason is that doctors were as a group behaving corruptly through the 1960s to 1980s where there was little oversight but healthcare spending grew strongly as doctors had more and more successful treatments available.(63) Medical doctors as a group engaged in widespread overservicing, performing unnecessary procedures and were wildly inefficient. That led to those who directly paid for medical care to attempt to rein in spending by taking more control of healthcare spending and of doctors themselves.

There are also deeper reasons apart from the above corruption as to why something as harmful as misused evidence-based medicine could control and disempower doctors.

It is a large and controversial statement to present that one of the main methods to decrease population health has been evidence-based medicine, but that is actually what is happening.

How did evidence-based medicine reduce population health? By stifling doctors and forcing them to engage in a process – evidence-based medicine – where every step of that process has been corrupted by vested interests that are able to act in unconscionable ways with very little if any hindrance.

One important aspect of evidence-based medicine as it is practised is that it considers doctors of comparable demographics to be interchangeable. What matters is the skill with which they apply guidelines, and most doctors have the skills to do that.

It is not true that doctors are interchangeable. Medical doctors make a big difference for their patients beyond the application of guidelines despite all the restrictions on their freedom to make decisions as my and other recent research has shown. (64-67) Yes, doctors may make many mistakes but during the heyday of medical doctors' independence and growth in successful treatments in the 1960s to 1980s, life expectancy rose substantially.

In theory, an empowered and efficient body of healthcare providers therefore may avoid most of the pitfalls of both evidence-based medicine and spiralling healthcare costs, but we are far from such a situation.

There are other reasons for the healthcare catastrophe we are witnessing now with healthcare getting more and more expensive just to manage the deterioration in health and rise in chronic diseases but one of the main reasons is how evidence-based medicine and other measures interfere with the doctors' ability to diagnose and to apply medical treatments.

For guidelines to assume supremacy, evidence-based medicine needs to assume that doctors with similar demographics such as training and experience are interchangeable. That is clearly not a correct assumption in the eyes of many or most patients. Many patients and their families will go to lengths to find a good or even the best doctor for a significant procedure or for a diagnosis that other doctors have failed to make. As evidence-based medicine is no help for those who take multiple medicines, which seems to be a majority of older people, doctors are at least equal to the guidelines, i.e. the implementation of evidence-based medicine.

If it is not true that doctors are interchangeable, is there published research that shows and confirms what everyone knows, which is that doctors actually make a difference to patients' physical health apart from applying guidelines for diagnostics and treatments?

The answer is yes, there is and has been since 2022. In 2022, two systematic reviews were published as part of my PhD.(64, 65). These publications showed that doctors make a difference to patients' physical health even after accounting for all known factors such as demographics and patient risk factors. That effect means that doctors have a healing ability that goes beyond applying guidelines for diagnostics and interventions (medical treatments). That doctors' effect has long been labelled as the placebo effect, an effect whose cause was unknown. Part or all of that placebo effect is the doctors' effect as defined above.

These healing abilities differ between doctors and, as an important detail, the exceptionally good doctors are not formally identified, even though that is possible; there is no systematic process to learn from them; and they are just as likely to be vilified as to be praised as they show patients what is possible, making those patients more demanding and exposing their colleagues.(68)

Also, in 2022 a seminal economics paper(66) was published showing conclusively that Norwegian GPs affect the life expectancy of their older patients substantially, either subtracting (the bottom 5%) or adding (the top 5%) an estimated nine months in life expectancy on average for each of their patients aged 55+ while being cheaper for the healthcare systems. Further, the bottom 5% had a 12.2% higher 2-year mortality rate and the top 5% a 12.2% lower mortality rate than the average doctor. Interestingly, the effectiveness of a GP in terms of life expectancy is almost uncorrelated with patients' rating and all the information the researchers had about the GPs and patients did not explain the difference between GPs.

A profession that does not use or is even aware of who their best members are and is making no moves to find out is a profession that has no authoritative clinicians. There are plenty of doctors who receive many medical research accolades but there are no clinicians known to the general public who can speak for the profession of the doctors who treat patients. Those who do speak and have a platform, have generally received their authorisation from external agencies such as the media or through senior administrative positions or through publishing widely cited research papers.

However, as shown during COVID-19, doctors with a very prestigious background in research were widely attacked by the media when their publications or opinions were against the prevailing narrative, regardless of the significance of their previous research.(69-72)

As a consequence, there are no doctors who are clinicians with authority to speak for their profession, with that authority derived from their clinical ability and not from other sources. As a consequence of this lack of authority, other parties such as health administrators, legislators, insurers etc can control the medical profession.

So, how do doctors and the world deal with the fact that doctors are the most successful healers on the planet as, in addition to their innate ability to heal, they have a plethora of tools, experience and, despite the corruption, knowledge available to maximise their effect?

Most doctors do not like the idea of being called healers but if you deny you are a healer, you deny an important part of your medical ability and you deny and thereby lose a substantial part of your ability as a clinician as your only authority is your level of knowledge, sometimes your physical skills and the authority given to you by external agencies and the amount of medical resources you control. Apart from any ownership of assets, each of these authorities can be taken away from you regardless of your clinical abilities. You lose an ability doctors from the previous century had, which was to speak from your own authority when giving advice to the patient.

If you only speak from knowledge and guidelines, then the patient can challenge what you say by finding alternative knowledge and guidelines. If you speak from personal authority as a person or clinician, the patient can still reject what you recommend but your statements will have an impact the patient may take up in future.

The research literature is instructive. Highly cited books and articles from last century(73, 74) often talk about paternalism and its abuse, while more current articles highlight the lack of authority that doctors now have, for example(75) stating that the patient should not be contradicted as that would affect the doctor-patient relationship. A 2011 paper highlights that 'patient-centredness' has little if any effect on patients' health outcomes.(76) Authority can be and has been abused by doctors but disempowering doctors does not make patients healthier. The newer research I found does not seem to be aware that doctors today have less authority than they did last century.

As regulators, administrators and evidence-based medicine in general consider a doctor to be largely replaceable by another doctor with similar demographics and are not even consciously aware that some doctors are inherently more capable than others as shown in a dialogue on an evidence-based mailing list(77) that is only available by subscription, they ignore doctors' healing ability, apart from seeking to identify and remove the worst performers.

In many ways it made no sense for the church in the Middle Ages to kill healers and thereby keep the population substantially sicker and less productive than would otherwise be the case but that is what happened and was maintained for centuries with only priests allowed to practise medicine.

A lot of explanations can be given to explain the motivations behind such sustainable harm, but one consideration is that these persecutions are about as far away from the central message of Christianity of love as one could possibly go by taking actions that diminish the entire population's health.

Persecuting healers in the Middle Ages made little sense but was engaged in with a lot of zeal. The church's ability to keep the health of their subject poor appeared to be important for the church.

The recent COVID-19 episode clearly shows that the powers that be are still strongly motivated to substantially worsening population health by using force and manipulation to inject healthy people with more than a billion doses(41, 42) of agents that damage their immune system.(46-50)

The powers that be, whoever they are, controlled and likely still control the vast majority of rich countries' and some or many poorer countries' politicians, regulators, media and public opinion that supported and support a measure that transparently damaged population health. This statement will be supported in detail later on.

Hence, as this level of control was used to cause harm to population health, it makes sense for those forces to reduce the impact of one of the strongest opposing forces that are against damaging population health on this planet – a substantial proportion of medical doctors.

Many medical doctors start out with or have a deep love of humanity and go through the arduous process of becoming doctors in order to improve people's health. Judging from what has actually been happening, which is a vast increase in doctors' ability to heal through more and more successful interventions and diagnostic tools, something else had to happen in order to manage population health in such a way that population health would not actually improve despite this massive growth in the capability and availability of healing tools and the reduction of smoking.

The groundwork to offset the increasing benefits of doctors was laid in the 1960s and 1970s by allowing many doctors to behave corruptly in giving them much more money without oversight, leading to an explosion in costs and unnecessary interventions.

This obvious corruption and wastage were then used by regulators to control spending and thereby diagnostic and treatment choices by doctors through accreditation requirements from health insurers, government regulators and, in the United States, managed care and health maintenance organisations and, especially through evidence-based medicine.

The Methods of Evidence-based Medicine

One feature of evidence-based medicine is that its research methods were misused to dissipate false truths that led to dramatic declines in population health.

A good example are the trials in the 1960s and 1970s that showed that cholesterol can be reduced by replacing more expensive animal fats with plant-based fats(78, 79) and, as a corollary, reducing fats in the diet altogether. Those same trials were reanalysed in 2013 and 2016(80, 81) and then showed that *increased* cholesterol linearly (the relationship is a straight line) <u>reduces</u> mortality and *decreased* cholesterol <u>increases</u> mortality, the opposite of the common assumption that more cholesterol is either bad for you or a sign of vascular or heart issues.

As a consequence of the two trials in the 1960s and 1970s, food companies and regulators had scientific backing to replace expensive fats with much cheaper sugar in order for food to still taste good.

Excess sugar seems to be the main dietary mechanism for obesity as eating sugar raises the blood sugar levels, leading to a feeling of satiation, leading to the liver storing the excess sugar as fat, leading to lower blood sugar levels and the desire to eat again. If that next meal is sugar or starch again, the same cycle continues.(82-84)

One consequence of overconsumption of sugar is the still rising obesity epidemic and the massive rise in chronic diseases, offsetting the benefits of any individual treatment such as treatments that have been able to reduce cancer mortality by 50%.(85)

Everything that has been happening for the last 100 years becomes a coherent whole under the assumption of a strong force working to make people sicker and sicker despite rapid scientific progress and the efforts of many doctors and other people who are working on improving population health. It is a preposterous assumption as there is no beneficiary except for those who advocate that a lower world population is better for the planet, but this is what actually happens. The first step in any diagnosis is to know what actually happened.

Also, it makes little sense to say that there is a force that controls most politicians, even more regulators and almost the entire media except for the fact that this is what actually happened from 2020 to 2023. Many of these people made and maintained statements that were transparently untrue even when presented with facts. The process of damaging population health was suddenly in everyone's face and very much out in the open.

There is no way to explain who was ultimately in charge of what happened with the information currently at hand but this co-ordinated assault on the world's population health has happened and it simply means that there are goings-on in this world we are not fully aware of. Blaming those who implemented these measures such as the gain-of-function researchers financed by the United States National Institute of Health (NIH) through NIAID,(24) or those who groomed some of the worst politicians such as the World Economic Forum(86) or the opportunism and control exercised by pharmaceutical companies is nowhere near adequate in explaining the worldwide co-ordination and control of the measures taken.

This book is not about speculating what those forces are but to put the last 100 years of medical treatments in context and to cover the global catastrophe in terms of impact on population health that evidence-based medicine is.

It is liberating to see what is happening as that clarity allows each individual to take, or not to take, any measures that are within their powers to act upon. Providing that clarity and empowering people and doctors is the purpose of this book. The book is an offer for us to open our eyes to what is actually happening and to take responsibility, starting from our own bodies.

CHAPTER 2

PEOPLE AND EVIDENCE-BASED MEDICINE

Introduction

People on a population basis do not demand to be healthy. They demand to have a cure or a management of their ailment when they are not healthy and not for them to take responsibility for lifestyle change. People are ready to tolerate amazing levels of ill health if the only way for them to get better is by changing their lifestyle.

Even when they are diagnosed with a chronic lifestyle disease, on a population basis the people who improve their behaviour are balanced by those whose behaviour worsens.(87) Patients, on a population basis, may do the minimum of what they have to do but if there is a choice of treatment, such as between a pill and a change in lifestyle, then the great majority go for the pill, not for the needed change in their lifestyle, even if the pill has much less of a beneficial effect than the change in lifestyle.

Statins are a good example. They do not improve mortality.(88-90) Exercise and diet changes reduce heart failures by 50% and also mortality but people prefer statins.(91)

A population that behaves so irresponsibly and that has those specific demands for interventions will get what they ask for, with evidence-based medicine providing the philosophical and physical underpinning of this satisfying of population health demands, especially as treating chronic illnesses incurs very high costs and therefore the financial incentives for the providers are in synchronicity with the desires of the patients as both prefer long-term pharmaceutical treatments for chronic illnesses.

This should not distract from the many medicines and therapies that are needed, properly prescribed, working well and at times seem miraculous. The issue is that the goodwill generated from these medicines and therapies has been abused to such a degree that it is bankrupting health systems and damaging population health.

Evidence-based medicine is a method where even highly dangerous and poisonous medicines can be declared to be sufficiently improving health for them to be sold as medicines with many examples provided by Peter Gøtzsche.(60) Just how dangerous and poisonous depends on a second influence, the political will at the time.

Peter Gøtzsche's book came out in 2013. I have not discerned any changes that have occurred since his describing many mechanisms on how this Faustian pact (deal with the devil) is executed.

In terms of widely accepted actually poisonous measures, a good example are the mRNA injections labelled to be vaccines for COVID-19. Among the many strategies used in making them look better than they are, one stands out:

Any adverse reactions within the first 7 or, frequently, 14 or 21 days of the injection were and are added to the non-injected population, with an example *"considered unvaccinated if <14 days had elapsed since receipt of the first dose in the primary series of an mRNA or Janssen vaccine".(92-94)*

This strategy would allow an outright poison such as strychnine to be proven to have strong powers of preventing death: You give a dose of strychnine that kills half the patients in a week but you add the deaths to the population as an event that happened before the taking of the poison, as the effects of the first seven or more days of administering the dose are not considered to be due to the strychnine. You therefore have a lot of deaths, according to your reporting, among the group you are investigating, supposedly before they took the strychnine.

It sounds completely preposterous to do this but that is precisely what the procedure for vaccines has been for centuries – the first 7-21 days' health events are counted as pre-vaccine health events and the media faithfully followed that script. As there were a substantial number of deaths and injuries within 7, 14, and 21 days of taking the vaccine, it seemed as if the unvaccinated had a high death rate and the vaccinated a lower death rate, even though the opposite happened as a large proportion of vaccine injuries and deaths happened soon after the inoculation.

Coming back to the strychnine example, according to this statistical trick, administering strychnine looks like a saviour of protecting from sudden, agonising death when it is really the cause of the death.

As the rules of evidence-based medicine currently allow this complete misrepresentation of the facts when it comes to vaccines, dangerous poisons can legitimately be sold as vaccines, provided that a substantial proportion of the damage shows up within 7, 14, and 21 days of administering. It is so outrageous a lie that many people have trouble understanding this.

How mortality is assigned to vaccination status after vaccine administration

Vaccinated

Vaccine Adverse Effects Reporting System (VAERS) Covid-19 Vaccine reported deaths by days to onset

Reports of Death

source:openvaers.com

Date of injection   Days to Onset

Deaths added to unvaccinated   Deaths added to vaccinated

How the US government in the form of the national institute of health (NIH) defines vaccination status

Graph based on design provided by X user KBirb @birb_k April 19th, 2024, https://x.com/birb_k/status/1781040192247210013

If you follow the rules of evidence-based medicine – and many rules can be made up on the spot, such as the above rule – then you have the right to call your research results to be true results, no matter the actual truth. This construct has made pharmaceutical companies very rich, as many medicines with doubtful or non-existent efficacy and large side effects were approved and therefore profitable. These profits allow pharmaceutical companies to financially corrupt doctors, regulators and influence politicians and the media and therefore pharmaceutical companies are getting the political backing to sell more and more expensive and often useless treatments or charge extremely high amounts for medicines that actually work.(95-114)

This will continue until population health is so poor and mortality is so high that the customers and therefore the enablers put a stop to it, but that may be decades or, as it was in the Middle Ages, centuries away. It could also happen very soon as there is a lively battle going on between those who receive the benefits from the patients' irresponsibility such as money, and those who dislike this state of affairs. **Currently the perpetrators are in almost complete control and that can only change when the enablers, the population at large, put a stop to it.**

If you go to a medical doctor, you are very likely receiving 'evidence-based medicine' from this doctor as evidence-based medicine is either mandatory for the doctor or highly encouraged. In addition, many doctors are enthusiastic or at least in favour of the practice as it has provided substantial benefits in many individual cases.

Up until the 1990s, the knowledge the doctor used was mostly their own experience, supplemented by anecdotes, case studies and what was considered expert opinion.(63) With the explosion of medical research being conducted since the 1970s it seemed by the 1990s that it was time to systematically add research results to the medical knowledge base. The reason is that research results in many cases were more objective or accurate than the opinion of individuals and it could be shown that many established medical practices could be substituted by practices that had better patient outcomes.(17, 115-117)

This process of adding medical research results to medical practice was labelled as *"evidence-based medicine"*(1, 118) and its title implied that this is a better approach than the then prevailing *"experience or opinion-based medicine"*.(119)

There were numerous instances where evidence-based medicine showed that the then current practice was inferior, sometimes wildly inferior to alternative methods.(119) It therefore made sense to assume that evidence-based medicine would lead to better population health outcomes.(120, 121)

And they happened. From 2000 to 2023, the chances of dying from a cancer one has been diagnosed with dropped by 50%. This benefit happened concurrently with the number of cancer diagnoses increasing by 34% most likely due to population aging as older people have more cancers.(85, 122)

However, other statistics worsened or did not improve beyond the rate they were already improving:

After 30 years, by 2024, evidence-based medicine, despite its widespread adoption, did not improve life expectancy beyond the rate of improvement already happening. In fact, despite millions of research papers, life expectancy in some countries is now reducing. Either there are other substantial influences negatively affecting population health and life expectancy or more medical research does not improve population health.

One component of the lack of population health benefit from evidence-based medicine is the research method it uses. The research method itself is neutral. When used without manipulation the research method can be used to acquire new knowledge for the party doing the research. That knowledge can then be used or misused. The research method can also be manipulated so that the desired result can be reported.

A good example for both is that evidence-based medicine can be considered to be one of the main agents responsible for the obesity epidemic as research results from the 1960s were used to substitute animal fats in the diet with plant-based fats and the much cheaper sugar,(123) with excess sugar being a likely contributor to weight gain.(82, 84, 124, 125)

Add to that food and beverage companies' extensive research to find foods and food ingredients that are hard to resist for humans and you end up with a population that permanently overeats, eats wrongly and gains weight at an accelerating rate.(126) This is an example of medical research benefitting organisations while harming the population. Part of the weight gain is associated with ceasing smoking(127) but levels of obesity are also increasing in those who never smoked and, as an example, the later a woman's year of birth, the more she has put on weight at a given age, i.e. the younger they are the more quickly they (we) put on weight on a population basis.(21)

Further, medical costs have substantially increased as a percentage of GDP, i.e. we are spending more and more per person on healthcare but do not get better results, with the United States spending the most on healthcare and therefore using the most evidence-based medicine but having one of the worst population health outcomes among wealthy nations.(9-14)

It would be interesting to investigate how much of the blowout in United States healthcare costs is due to the emphasis on specialist care rather than primary care, how much is due to the quantity of pharmaceuticals consumed (a direct consequence of using research methods that are part of evidence-based medicine) and how much is due to an overall worse level of population health.

There is a circularity between consumption levels of pharmaceuticals and bad health,(60, 128) the lack of emphasis on primary care(129-132) and bad health, the level of quality in food eaten and bad health,(95, 133) with evidence-based medicine as stated directly responsible for at least one aspect of that bad food quality with its emphasis against fats in food and in favour of sugar.(80, 81, 84, 123, 125, 126)

In other words, unlike other healthcare measures such as sanitations including flushing toilets and other hygiene methods such as using disinfectants intelligently, evidence-based medicine seems to be either an expensive non-event or even detrimental to population health, notwithstanding that individuals are at times deriving huge health benefits from medical research,(17, 116, 117, 134) such as in treatments of heart attacks and strokes,(115, 135) but that is not the whole story.

The Harm of Evidence-based Medicine

That overall non-progress or decline in life expectancy need not be due to evidence-based medicine as other influences could be depressing population health, though the evidence-based medicine associated harms have increased over time, reaching a crescendo in the COVID-19 creation and response. These harms are intrinsic to the design of evidence-based medicine.

These harms are also intrinsic to medical research in general even if there is medical research that is not evidence-based medicine as the benefits of tipping the scales in medical research for the researcher and the sponsor and the future job prospects of the regulators are so extraordinarily large. Medical research can and will be corrupted. The key is our response to that corruption. At the moment, corrupt behaviour is career enhancing and only in its most egregious violations is there a possibility of it being called out, and that is after the harm has been done.(136-139)

There are ways to deal with the harm of evidence-based medicine, such as making doctors at least an equal in standing to guidelines and tight, effective controls on conflicts of interests in those who write guidelines, but those ways are not even considered by the healthcare experts and authorities at the moment and the ways that are considered – tightening research standards, and increasing controls and medical regulations – make things worse by making research more expensive.

It may also be practically very difficult or impossible to find unconflicted guideline writers where substantial healthcare spending is influenced by the guidelines as there are plenty of non-monetary means of influencing people by rewarding those the targets care about, by perfectly legally lobbying those who have an influence on those writing guidelines, etc.

In the early years, i.e. 1990s and early 2000s, evidence-based medicine provided research results that were of limited use in clinical practice and required commitment by medical practitioners to keep up with research developments(140, 141) and the at times contradictory results from medical research.(142) All of these issues were seemingly handled by the creation of authoritative guidelines, after some initial hiccups,(143) the establishment of these guidelines had consequences:

a. Every step in the creation of these guidelines can be corrupted.(97-104, 106-111, 113, 144-147) Disclosure of conflicts of interest(96) need not work and does not work(148) as those who evaluate the level of conflict can be corrupt and the question arises why there should be an obvious conflict at all?

b. Doctors lost a tremendous amount of power and flexibility in clinical practice as the burden of proof is now on them(149) if they do not follow authoritative guidelines and insurance reimbursements can be tied to complying with guidelines.

    This disempowerment of doctors and neglect of research on doctors' contributions to patients' health has gone so far that until 2022 there was no systematic research to establish whether doctors make a difference to patients' physical health by themselves, i.e. after all known information is considered and beyond demographic characteristics such as experience and education.(64, 65, 150) In other words, on a research basis, there was no evidence that doctors make a difference beyond their experience and level of education and therefore they had and in practice still have no authority as medical doctors beyond the authority given by their license, their education and their experience. Consequently doctors are considered replaceable by somebody temporally equally qualified.

In fact, there is a prevalent opinion among evidence-based medical researchers that most of the time doctors make no difference to their patients' health as they follow guidelines for diagnostics and interventions (treatments) as shown in a dialogue on an evidence-based medicine mailing list.(77)

In practice the fact that guidelines have limited or no application or can be plain wrong when dealing with multi-symptomatic people,(120) leaving the disempowered doctor on their own, this fact is simply ignored in clinical practice.

c. Evidence-based medicine favours medical research results that follow certain rules. These research results can be and are extensively manipulated by interested parties leading to the evidence used being partly or completely falsified. Lies that benefit interest groups are accepted as truths.(97, 99-103, 106-108)

d. The authors of guidelines can and do have extensive conflicts of interest, further falsifying the research results that are used to justify the practices recommended by the guidelines.(96-98, 108)

e. Evidence-based medicine is of very limited use in the majority of patients as these patients are multi-symptomatic and it is practically impossible to research more than a few combinations of medicines that are taken simultaneously for multiple treatments. There is no research evidence for a person who takes 4, 5, 10, or 20 different medications. The doctor is completely on their own.(120)

f. Evidence-based medicine in practice narrowly focuses on one part of the medical interaction, the intervention, and then provides in many cases deeply flawed evidence for its favoured interventions. That is the case even though more than a billion medical interactions each year(151, 152) consists at least of a doctor, a patient, and an intervention. The doctor is considered little more than a highly qualified employer of guidelines. The patient is rarely asked to behave responsibly and thereby support the healing process, for example by simply following a treatment plan.

CHAPTER 3

GUIDELINES

Evidence-based Medicine and Guidelines

As mentioned, in 1999, David Sackett, an epidemiologist, made a very famous statement that read as follows:

> *"[T]he practice of evidence-based medicine means integrating individual clinical expertise with a critical appraisal of the best available external clinical evidence from systematic research."(1)*

This seemingly obvious and entirely unobjectionable statement has led to the current global catastrophe in population health as *"the best available external clinical evidence from systematic research"* became guidelines.

Ignoring guidelines is difficult or dangerous for a medical doctor as they can be mandatory. Ignoring guidelines exposes doctors to lawsuits when the patient takes a turn for the worse or can lead to intervention by employers, regulators, or medical tribunals.

Guidelines have tremendous authority, in many cases more authority than the individual doctor.

Guidelines in the worst cases can be mandated by authorities even if they lead to millions of deaths and are clearly not based on evidence such as for the diagnosis and treatment of COVID-19 where working and safe pharmaceutical treatments were rejected despite there being a long-term systematic review of such treatments(153) in favour of treatments that harmed more than they worked or were much less effective, such as remdesivir, paxlovid and molnuparivir(154-156) and diagnostic tests were mandated that were unsuitable.(157, 158)

Guidelines are manipulated in many different ways.(159) Some of them include:

Authors of guidelines can be compromised due to conflicts of interests leading to guidelines that do not favour the best treatment or limit medical doctors' choices but benefit the sponsor of those authors.

Guidelines can be compromised by manipulating the "*best available clinical evidence*" by influencing or outright fabricating "*systematic research*" and the medical trials that are analysed in systematic research.

Blatant cases like COVID-19 where guidelines are used that clearly go against the evidence may (or may not) be relatively rare but influenced or fabricated systematic research is very common(160, 161) and has caused tremendous harm to population health.(146, 162)

Guidelines came about because in the early 2000s there were a lot of people pointing out the practical difficulties inherent in the words *"best available external clinical evidence "*(1) with the below as a good example:

> *"Nowhere in the EBM process is listening to patients and their concerns, and legitimizing their questions, regarded as important."(163)*

> *"In the sense that the voice of the patient is explicitly excluded in the steps of EBM, except insofar as it is a voice of pathological information that can be transformed into searchable terms, it is no wonder that proponents of EBM can still write of the problematic nature of including patient values and perspectives (see, for example, Haynes 2002(164)). They are omitted from the process by definition."(163)*

> *"The paradox here is that evidence is created and generated from a group of people that is quite different from the group of people where it is applied. The context of discovery, as it were, is markedly different from the context of application.*

> *This causes conceptual problems for strict evidence-based approaches to medicine. It also raises issues about what kind of warrant a clinical trial provides for making treatment recommendations when embarking on paths of care. Insufficient attention has been paid to the issue of when extrapolations from the strict inclusion and exclusion criteria are*

appropriate. These extrapolations occur frequently in clinical medicine and have unclear sanction in the universe of EBM. Such extrapolations also highlight the tolerance of a peculiar "inference gap" within the theory of EBM, about which more below.

The issue also illustrates out how poorly we understand exactly what the results of any clinical trial mean. As Richard Horton (2000)(165) has written that "issues of external validity are the most important that face clinical research today and that the failure to resolve them is largely responsible for the indifference doctors world wide show towards research evidence." Clinical research evidence in the form of RCTs and meta-analyses provides at best a provisional warrant—that is, drug X may work, not drug X will work. The probability of successful treatment with the assortment of agents available varies dramatically; there is a wide range of ways of framing these benefits, but there is no such thing as a treatment that works every time. Consequently, there is nothing in any way directive about such evidence and nothing inevitable about a p value or confidence interval: the evidence does not tell a physician or a patient what to do and has no compelling epistemic or moral force."(163)

"Unfortunately, I live in a world where single problems and single therapies rarely present themselves. When one adds complexity to the mix, the number of possible options increases dramatically."(163)

The aim of evidence-based medicine was not to rely solely or mainly on the personal experience of the medical doctor but to combine that with objective evidence. This reliance on personal experience was scathingly referred to as 'GOBSAT' or Good Old Boys Sitting Around A Table by one of the popularisers of evidence-based medicine, Trisha Greenhalgh.(119) Professor Greenhalgh later expressed doubts about evidence-based medicine when she experienced those treatments on her own body.(120, 166)

As the addition of research-based evidence ran into the practical problems described above, the adopted solution turned out to be guidelines which happen to be put together by a more inclusive version of good old boys sitting around a table, except that these Gobsats now had authority, immensely simplifying the process for interested parties such as pharmaceutical companies to get doctors to behave in ways supportive to these interested parties as only a small number of Gobsats of any gender and colour needed to be influenced, steered, directed, 'supported', encouraged. Name any euphemism for what is pervasive corruption,(60, 91, 95-114, 128, 142, 167) as patient values are almost completely ignored.(168)

CHAPTER 4

DOCTORS AND EVIDENCE-BASED MEDICINE

The Disempowerment of Doctors

U p until the mid-1990s in many countries doctors were relatively free to exercise their clinical judgment even going against medical guidelines. *"ICSI adopted the rule used by Salt Lake City's LDS Hospital: if a doctor disregarded a guideline, the doctor was presumed right and the guideline wrong until it was shown otherwise."*(63) The ICSI (Institute for Clinical Systems Integration) is spin-off of the United States Business Health Care Action Group, a group of company representatives formed to reduce healthcare costs, a substantial proportion of which is covered by companies for their employees.

The main threat free to exercising clinical judgment was litigation and that mostly in the United States.

Since then it has become more and more problematic for doctors to provide care that is at variance of the guidelines as they may get into difficulties through litigation, regulators, and employers or even legislation as for example many places prohibited early stage treatments of COVID-19.(169-172)

Doctors allowed themselves to be considered replaceable and there was hardly any research by doctors or anybody else investigating whether doctors make a difference by themselves to patients' physical health – psychotherapists in contrast established that they make a substantial difference to their patients' mental health.(173) It was necessary for psychotherapists to do so because pharmaceuticals worked no better than placebos for the treatment of mental health except in the worst cases. Hence, unlike medical doctors, psychotherapists could not rely on the physical intervention to justify their existence and had to find another reason such as psychotherapists themselves making a difference.(173, 174)

What is the benefit for the doctor in being considered replaceable and being forced to follow guidelines and also being on their own for many of their patients, as there is no evidence on how to treat multi-symptomatic people and many remedies have never been tested for all relevant age groups or even had no randomised controlled trials at all such as in the case of vaccines?(23)

It is hard to make sense why a respected, important, and well-paid profession gave its power away to such a degree to guidelines, guidelines which its members know only apply to a subgroup of patients and leave the doctors with the worst of all worlds – no power, no guidelines – for the balance of their patients.

One possibility is that the medical profession was vulnerable to an external takeover. Medicine ran on a rigid hierarchy with specialists above generalists and seniority given authority, or *"Demi-Gods in White"* as chief hospital physicians were referred to in the German media in the 1970s and 1980s. Once scientific evidence came in showing that many established practices such as radical mastectomy were unnecessary or harmful,(134) or could be improved substantially(115, 116) these chief physicians lost authority. Another reason is that doctors abused the time where there was little oversight by overcharging, over-diagnosing and over-treating, leading to an urgent need for those financing healthcare to introduce financial and then more intrusive controls which affected medical professionals.(63) It seems that doctors still perceived a need for an external authority and that authority was assumed by medical guidelines. The disastrous confluence of submitting to this external authority with massive levels of burnout,(175-183) poor population health(21, 120, 184-186) and large healthcare costs may require a rethink.

In contrast, pharmaceutical companies through intense lobbying of government and financing the media in the United States, doctors and researchers made sure that on balance the extra levels of control either benefited them or only affected them in limited ways.

Pharmaceutical companies benefit from the commonly in research adopted CONSORT guidelines(187) on reporting trials as these made clinical trials more expensive, giving those with more funds more control on what to fund and reduce research they do not favour.

Lobbying had the consequence that United States Medicare was not allowed to negotiate prices with pharmaceutical companies until 2022.(188, 189)

Any harm to pharmaceutical companies in the form of even multi-billion dollar fines were kept in perspective as the profits from the transgressions often dwarfed even the biggest fines.(60)

Giving authority to medical guidelines has consequences. It leads in practice to the thinking that doctors do not matter beyond their knowledge and ability to apply medical guidelines as this example shows:

> *"Of course, without a practitioner and a patient, no clinical encounter can happen. My point was that most of the time (9 of 10, 99 of 100 – I don't know), it does not matter if the patient is seen by you, me, or someone else (as long as delivery of health services adhered to EBM recommendations that often can be algorithmically implemented). Yes, in some rare (or, not so rare?) circumstances patients' outcomes will be hugely affected by the practitioners' skills."(77)*

This was written by Benjamin Djulbegovic,(190) a highly respected expert on evidence-based medicine who is also a trained medical doctor (MD) and professor of medicine whose scientific publications had received 52,200 citations by early 2024 and who has an h-index of 80 on Google and a very high h-index of 69 on Scopus, a medical database, i.e. 80 (69) publications with at least 80 (69) citations each, making him one of the most-cited medical researchers in the world, and his above expressed opinion seems to be the prevailing view among adherents of evidence-based medicine.

Do Doctors Themselves Make A Difference to Patients' Physical Health Beyond Diagnostics and Intervention?

If that outlook is true that the choice of doctor most or almost all of the time does not matter, doctors are replaceable and the guidelines are what matters.

However, that statement is not true. Doctors make a difference to patients' physical health.

Depending on what is measured and what the intervention is, that difference that doctors make can be negligible (anaesthetists' influence on patient mortality is an example, though anaesthetists may have a large influence on post operative pain experienced by the patient) to a doctors' effect that is very large, dwarfing the effect of most interventions, for example shoulder surgery.(64, 65)

This fact came out of the investigations of the author as part of his PhD on "*What makes an exceptionally good doctor*" and doctor performance in general. Up to my publications from 2022 onwards and a fascinating economics paper(66) in the same year there was no answer to whether doctors make a difference to patients' physical health beyond all known factors, in the scientific literature. One reason for this surprising lack of interest could be that doctors through the rise of evidence-based medicine can successfully avoid ever being labelled as healers and can only be considered to be highly qualified technicians with communications and empathy being parts of the technicians' (i.e. medical doctors') skillset.

If doctors make a difference to patients' physical health – and they do – then that means that their performance differs. The reason is as follows:

If every doctor has the same effect on patients' physical health, after accounting for demographic factors such as training and experience, and if that effect is measurable, then it can be found by comparing patients' health outcomes with patients who do not receive medical treatment or treatment from other clinicians. In that case doctors are interchangeable with doctors with the same relevant demographics.

If doctors have an effect beyond their demographics and their performance differs, then in multi-level statistics doctors are responsible for part of the variation in patients' physical health outcomes and that part can be measured. It turned out that that part can range from negligible to very large. In reverse, if there is variation in patients' physical health outcomes, then some doctors have better or worse (different) results to other doctors that go beyond random fluctuations. As there are doctors whose performance is statistically significantly superior to that of their brethren, such doctors have a valuable ability to share.

It is well established that there are bad doctors but until the author's research it was not at all established that there are exceptionally good doctors(64-66, 191, 192) and, more importantly, that they can be identified by analysing medical records,(64-66, 150) with the exception of one non-peer-reviewed economics paper.(67) It also was not established that doctors have an influence on patients' physical health even after accounting for all known information such as doctor experience and education and patient risk factors. In other words, there are better and worse doctors and by that fact not being scientifically established, doctors are only required to not be among the worst of their peers but are not required to identify and learn from the best, as officially nobody knows who the best doctors are.(77)

This stance of avoiding the responsibility of both systematically learning from their best brethren, and to acknowledge that doctors' ability is on a continuum ranging from the worst to the best is particularly surprising if we consider that **patients are very aware of these differences in quality and anybody the author knows who is about to undergo a dangerous procedure or has failed to receive a diagnosis from several doctors will go to substantial lengths to get the best doctor available.**

A recent search of the literature also found two very interesting papers, with the first(66) from 2022 showing conclusively that a better GP (family doctor) in Norway reduces the chance of a 55 or older patient dying within the next 2 years by 12.2%. The study covered all 5,000 Norwegian GPs and their 5.5 million patients of which 2,064 GPs fit the selection criteria. As governments put a value on achieving longer life for their citizens, in Norway a value of about $35,000 per healthy year of life added, each such better GP adds $9 million in value. The better doctor also reduces healthcare costs.

The second paper(67) from 2017 shows that the better hospital physicians in a teaching hospital consistently save an average

$2,000 or about 5% on treatment costs per patient and have better health outcomes.

The first paper(66) is very well researched and is able to show what is called 'causality'. Normally, in observational studies such as this which investigated Norwegian medical records, there could always be other reasons why one GP is better than another. A typical example is doctors in richer areas or with younger clients having a lower mortality. The researchers could eliminate those confounders because patients are randomly assigned to new doctors in the same town when a GP retires or reduces their workload.

It is difficult to overstate the importance of this paper. It shows that GPs make a very substantial difference to patients' health and most of that difference could not be explained by any doctor or patient data the researchers had access to. The authors concentrated on the financial benefit of bringing up the bottom 5% to average performance but the same value add applied for the top 5% doctors over the average doctor.

Hence it is equally valuable to learn from the best performers as it is to upskill the bottom performers.

A further interesting finding was that the doctors' performance on patients' mortality only affected patients' ratings in a very minor way. Patients in Norway were unable to discern how good or bad their doctor was in regard to the patients' mortality.

Clearly, there is a rich vein of research to mine here with doing qualitative studies of these Norwegian doctors to find out how the best doctors differ from the average doctor and the worst doctors being only the very start.

Consequences If Doctors Consider Themselves to be Highly Skilled Technicians

The *"I am not a healer but a skilled technician"* is heavily ingrained during medical school where facts reign supreme, where there is little training in communication and certainly no training to be a greater healer as it is not known what makes a greater healer among doctors as not even the concept of a doctor being a healer is discussed or considered. In fact, one way to make many doctors very uncomfortable is to state to them that they are healers. Typically, in my experience this statement gets quite vehemently denied.

Many doctors accept payments from pharmaceutical companies which alters their behaviour such as prescribing fewer generics and more on-patent pharmaceuticals. Many go further by accepting large payments and becoming spokespersons, formally or informally, for pharmaceutical companies and there are many examples such as in Peter Gøtzsche's book, of doctors behaving corruptly.(60)

One could expect that insurance reimbursements that differ between interventions would also modify many doctors' behaviour.

This behaviour can be called corrupt as it is harming for patients, but it can also be a form of conforming. If a doctor is corrupt and goes with the financial flow, they do not stand out and are in fact supported and promoted.

There are many doctors who do not go with the financial flow and would be expected to be better healers which is a reward in itself and can lead to a doctor being highly sought after but, as my research showed, such doctors are no more popular than the average doctor and are, as they do not necessarily follow the often corrupt guidelines or health insurance company directives, constantly under peer and regulatory pressure.

Going with the financial flow leads to a quieter life with good earnings though perhaps less job satisfaction and less purpose in life.

Eventually, though there is a price to pay for going along with measures that harm patients but are strongly demanded by external forces such as the media, regulators and legislators once the harm becomes obvious to patients, such as the COVID-19 measures where trust in physicians has substantially reduced from 72% to 40% in a large patient survey published in 2024.(193) I expect that such a reduction in trust will have extensive consequences for doctors unless they take steps to reverse that decline.

The selection of medical students and the training of doctors directly supports a tendency to go with the financial flow as the training is in many ways an extension of school years with a strong emphasis on acquiring huge amounts of knowledge(194-196) but very little understanding of healing and humans. This is exacerbated first by the sheer volume and prescriptiveness of learning and in doctors' first clinical years where it is very difficult not to come out completely exhausted, an exhaustion that can take years to overcome.(197-200) Medical education is also routinely and substantially influenced by pharmaceutical companies.(201, 202)

Such exploitation and control breeds disappointment, suppresses the desire to be of service and easily leads to cynicism and dishonesty.(203) Some doctors are able to resist this pressure but many doctors become burnt out. One harmful way to reduce the symptoms and exhaustion of burnout is to join the system, take the money and in extreme cases become a doctor who in their rage and disappointment knowingly and actively engages in activities that appear to benefit them, but are harmful for patients. Doctors who engage in gain-of-function research to create bioweapons are an extreme example.(23, 24)

Currently the training of doctors seems designed to breed exhaustion, cynicism and disappointment.(194-196, 204) That could easily be changed but that needed change, that many people can see is needed, is not happening. There is too much co-operation from medical students and junior doctors and patients who do not protest when their treating doctor is exhausted to reduce such egregious behaviour from their more senior peers, lecturers, legislators, financers and administrators.

Consider the madness in financial terms and in costs to human welfare to very expensively train large numbers of people in such a way that they drop out, change careers or work at a reduced capacity, i.e. part time or at lower effectiveness.

CHAPTER 5

PATIENTS

Introduction and Context

In David Sackett's original statement as a letter to the British Medical Journal (BMJ) in 1996 the patient is a recipient of measures decided by the doctor:

> *"Evidence based medicine is the conscientious, explicit, and judicious use of current best evidence in making decisions about the care of individual patients.*
>
> *The practice of evidence based medicine means integrating individual clinical expertise with the best available external clinical evidence from systematic research.*
>
> *By individual clinical expertise we mean the proficiency and judgment that individual clinicians acquire through clinical experience and clinical practice.*

*Increased expertise is reflected in many ways, but especially in more effective and efficient diagnosis and in the more thoughtful identification and compassionate use of individual **patients'** predicaments, rights, and preferences in making clinical decisions about their care.*

*By best available external clinical evidence we mean clinically relevant research, often from the basic sciences of medicine, but especially from **patient centred clinical research into the accuracy and precision of diagnostic tests (including the clinical examination), the power of prognostic markers, and the efficacy and safety of therapeutic, rehabilitative, and preventive regimens.**"(1)*

Every medical encounter that is the subject of this book consists of a doctor, a patient, and an intervention. The original impulse of evidence-based medicine has the patient as a recipient of the doctor's decisions, a mainly passive role. There have been substantial developments in including patients as active agents in the process but that is not part of the original impulse.

A more subtle point which is open to interpretation is that what is also missing is the doctor's intuition or opinion. The only item asked for from the doctor is individual clinical expertise and that "individual" part has been steadily reduced since 1996 by supplying guidelines for diagnosis and treatments.

Even though the doctor's 'individual clinical expertise' is originally half of the input of evidence-based medicine or equal to the evidence, there is comparatively very little research on this 'individual clinical expertise' and therefore on how that specific doctor in that particular encounter treats that particular patient.

Evidence-based medicine in its original impulse further covers only a very narrow part of the doctor/patient/intervention process as it only covers the doctor's clinical expertise and the evidence from systematic research and no other research such as case studies. It makes sense that when a narrow part of a process is emphasised at the expense of the rest of the process that that configuration leads to sub-optimal outcomes.

The whole concept of evidence-based medicine is fundamentally flawed as it disempowers doctors and empowers guidelines. Another big flaw is that, according to evidence-based medicine's philosophy, any statement that fulfils certain formal requirements is considered to be true until shown otherwise. In contrast, any doctor's action is considered to be potentially wrong unless shown otherwise by adhering to guidelines or shown to be in accord with external clinical evidence.

Another example is medical specialists. Specialists by definition have access to more external clinical evidence through their training and through their ability to limit their knowledge acquisition to a more confined area of medicine which they have the time to investigate more deeply, yet population health is determined by the level of primary care that is available and not by the level of specialist care.(131, 132, 205) A much poorer country can have substantially better health outcomes than a much richer country such as Slovenia vs United States.(206)

As one example of many, 60% of panel and taskforce members who developed the Diagnostic and Statistical Manual of Mental Disorders, fifth edition, text revision (DSM-5-TR) received $14.2m from industry – conflicts of interest among panel members that write guidelines are rife.(144-146, 207, 208)

Evidence-based Medicine and the Role of the Patient

At times, evidence-based medicine seems to miss an important point: When talking to a group of general practitioners (family medicine) doctors I was struck by the strength of their agreement to a remark of mine that many patients are quite irresponsible. In the doctors' experience many patients want to get a quick fix to their ailments and they do not want to make the necessary changes in their life to improve their health unless forced to,(87, 91) particularly when it comes to long-term conditions which can range from sleeplessness to multiple severe chronic illnesses.

Dealing with a large number of irresponsible people during the day puts a lot of pressure on doctors and could be a major contributor to the high levels of stress and burnout experienced by medical professionals as the ones who are most patient-facing in their work show the highest levels of stress and burnout.(175)

In other words, it seems that many patients do not want to hear what is best for them but want to get better with as little effort as possible on their part. Over the last decades, with an ageing population and the consequent rise in chronic conditions, this unwillingness on the part of patients to change their lifestyle but get fixed instead, looks as if it has become ever more common and the medical profession has been faced with a dilemma:

Doctors know what their patients need to do but the patients often do not want to implement what the doctors recommend or, even if the patients are responsible and have the intention to improve their life, they are then usually unable to sustain the changes they have started to implement,(209-212) although minor successes are possible.(213)

Evidence-based medicine comes to the seeming rescue in this situation. On the whole, evidence-based medicine allows the patient to receive an intervention, which may be a pharmacological or other treatment, without changing the way they live, because, due to evidence-based medicine, there is scientific evidence that this intervention works. How well does the intervention work? That seems to vary and is a question that will be discussed in detail later.

Evidence-based medicine also allows the doctor, through their experience, to quickly ascertain whether the patient is open to improve the way they live and, if not, to still do something that is helpful for them.

Instead of a doctor saying to a patient what they need to do in terms of lifestyle changes, the doctor can prescribe an intervention, which can be a pill or a treatment plan. Few interventions for chronic diseases and their acute consequences work as well as lifestyle changes do with many examples given in this book(91) but the evidence-based medical intervention is the next best option available after the patient has rejected the best available remedy, improving the way they live.

The evidence-based medical intervention has another big advantage in that it can be given in the typical 6-15 minute consultancy while a talk on lifestyle changes would be difficult to provide in such a short time span.

The trouble is that both doctor and patient are behaving irresponsibly in this exchange, and, over time, the accumulation of these irresponsible actions has dire consequences.

Patients get better treatments compared to receiving no treatment but overall, we are, for example, unable to stem the rising levels of obesity and its consequences and the cases of cancer, reported at an increasing rate(214) with the Australian age-standardised rate per 100,000 rising by 26% from 383.2 in 1982 to 483.8 in 2014, which, together with an ageing population, means that we have more and more cancer cases, as older people also get many more cancers than younger people.

Also, our chance of getting cancer has risen by 26% in 32 years or by ¾ of a percent every year, regardless of our age. This means that even the odds of young people to get cancer have been rising every year. That is a worrying development, especially as during that time smoking, which is a large cause of cancer, became less and less common. The raw (not standardised by age) rate per 100,000 increased by 34% in the United States from 2000 to 2023.(85, 122) There is currently also a lot of anecdotal evidence that since COVID-19 there has been another large increase in mortality(51, 52, 215), mental health issues(216) and dementia(217) with many pointing at the mRNA vaccines as being causative.

Cancer cases also seem to be on the increase with one cause given as reduced screening, diagnosis and treatment during the pandemic.(218)

Patients are more likely now to survive cancer with the mortality-to-incidence ratio, i.e. your chance of dying from that cancer when you have been diagnosed, dropping from 55% to 34%,(ibid.) though more people get cancer, negating half the benefit of evidence-based medicine due to a 26% increase in diagnosed cancers.

For doctors, the consequences of evidence-based medicine are becoming more and more apparent(120): By replacing their own clinical judgment and intuition with a set of rules, they disempower themselves as their authority is not theirs any more but an authority borrowed from an external source.

Evidence-based medicine is a tool. It is an incredibly useful tool when used well(17, 115-117, 219) and it is harmful and oppressive and very poor value for money when it is misused.(60, 91, 120) The basic difficulty with evidence-based medicine is that it creates very strong incentives to misuse it. Evidence-based medicine is rules-based and rules can be gamed, i.e. manipulated to one's advantage.(162, 220-222)

Patients can be extremely tolerant of being harmed through medication if they experience a need for that medication. When the COVID-19 vaccinations in Australia happened, people who were hospitalised after the first injection still took, on the advice of their doctors the second injection especially if they wanted to travel. After a while, everyone I asked knew multiple people who were severely ill after vaccination but a number of them still chose to take boosters. One anecdote described a long queue in front of a vaccination site and one person was taken out on a stretcher past the queue. Few, if any left that queue.

CHAPTER 6

EVIDENCE-BASED MEDICINE IN ACTION – CORRUPTION AT EVERY LEVEL:
COVID-19, IVERMECTIN, HYDROXYCHLOROQUINE AND NEWLY DEVELOPED REMEDIES

The Origin of COVID-19 – From Bat via Pangolin (An Animal) To Human or Through Biological Warfare and Lab Leak or Lab Release?

The United States National Institutes of Health (NIH), *"the nation's medical research agency"*(223) through its National-al Institute of Allergy and Infectious Diseases (NIAID) under the long term leader Anthony Fauci supported research in making pathogens more dangerous by making them easier to spread or making them more physically harmful to humans.

The reason given was to develop treatments.

This begs the question what the net benefit would be from such research except to conduct biological warfare while at best protecting one's own population if a good vaccine was developed in parallel. This research was labelled gain-of-function and part of that research was stopped in the United States in 2014 by declaring a moratorium with the following references reporting or commenting on the NIH funding gain-of-function research.(23-38)

The NIAID responded by funding EcoHealth Alliance, a United States non-profit that forwarded part of the funding to the Wuhan Institute of Virology in China, to continue with the research that was forbidden in the United States. There are copious records of these activities, documented in an overview here.(25)

In 2019, a new respiratory coronavirus was found in Wuhan with the most cited (5,350 Google citations) claiming its origin being from animals (zoonotic)(224) and reinforced by other published research.(225, 226) The simple thesis that a virus originating in the same city as a research institute conducting research into how to make respiratory viruses more lethal and contagious has been discounted heavily in prestigious scientific journals such as Science(225-227) while being supported initially by fringe publications(25, 228, 229) and later by newspapers such as The New York Times,(230) the UK Sunday Times and The Times.(26, 27) A summary of the evidence was published in 2023 in the British Medical Journal(28) and here(231) and a forceful rebuttal here.(232) Robert F. Kennedy Jr wrote a very detailed book about the strategies and methods used to hide the origin of the virus.(24)

Hence, there is clear evidence that research exists to make viruses more dangerous, and a new, seemingly dangerous pathogen was isolated near a laboratory that engaged in such research. Occam's razor(233) *"of two competing theories, the simpler explanation of an entity is to be preferred"* points to a lab leak.

This was confirmed by a December, 2024 report by the Select Subcommittee on the Coronavirus Pandemic Committee on Oversight and Accountability which states on page one *"SARS-CoV-2, the Virus that Causes COVID-19, Likely Emerged Because of a Laboratory or Research Related Accident."*(234)

A lot of people consider the facts of the United States and Chinese government supporting research to make viruses more virulent and lethal to be morally outrageous and have written detailed summaries of varying but at times high quality.(23, 231, 235-237) The usual argument is having to be prepared for what your enemies could do and that it is important to study lethal viruses – which already exist, such as Ebola and Marburg – or to study lethal respiratory viruses in order to be prepared for a pandemic with remedies such as the 1918 pandemic or that there is a benefit in being able to spread lethal viruses among your enemies while protecting your own population through vaccination.

This is evidence-based medicine in action, here used to deliberately cause maximum harm.

It is also an example of two countries who may come to blows in future jointly engaging in activities that harm their populations. On the face of it such actions of co-operating with a likely future enemy against your own people make little sense unless both conspire against a third country which in the current context also makes no sense. In fact, none of this makes any human sense.

These arguments for gain-of-function research are either wildly destructive or utterly stupid as viruses can and do leak from laboratories and thereby cause a lethal pandemic before counter measures are found.

COVID-19 was not one such event as the virus, with conservative treatment, was no more lethal than a bad flu and because there are, in addition, multiple very successful treatments and prevention strategies available as shown on this ongoing systematic review of 50+ treatments.(40)

As it turned out, COVID-19 is one of the easiest viral diseases ever to treat(236) as there are so many successful treatments for each stage available(153, 238) but, as shown later, with the evidence of the simplicity and effectiveness of antiviral agents being suppressed, the whole world was put through what amounted to a dress rehearsal of a lethal pandemic with lockdowns, social distancing, masks,(55) forced vaccinations, restrictive new legislation and the substantial harmful consequences of these measures.(53, 54)

The naming of COVID-19

Up to 2020, respiratory virus epidemics were named after their estimated physical origin or after the original host, such as the Hong Kong flu, Spanish flu, or Swine flu. In the same tradition, Sars COVID-19 would have been called the Wuhan virus.

However, the International Committee on Taxonomy of Viruses (ICTV)(239) preferred to use the labels coronavirus disease (COVID-19), with '19' standing for 2019, the year of first discovery, and to call the virus *"severe acute respiratory syndrome coronavirus 2 (SARS-CoV-2)"* with no mention of its origin in the name.

One Arm of Evidence-based Medicine Is Biological Warfare, The Perversion of the Scientific Method in Medical Research, and Its History

In 1859, Charles Darwin published his book "On the Origin of Species" with its central idea of the survival of the fittest. This idea was expanded by his second cousin Francis Galton,(240) who was instrumental in developing many scientific concepts such as regression, correlation, biometrics, fingerprints and genetics. Galton also coined the term eugenics, coming from the Greek "good in birth" as an extension of Darwin's survival of the fittest theory onto humanity by improving the human genetic stock through selective breeding. One of the main tools of selective breeding was sterilising and later wholesale killing of humans deemed to be less desirable. This was made clearer in the term *"racial hygiene"*, which was used interchangeably with eugenics.(241, pg 109)

By the turn of the century, this idea gained wide circulation in the United States, leading to 30 states passing sterilisation laws between 1907 and 1931 with 19 states still having such statutes on their books in 1987(242) and was supported by wealthy philanthropists such as the Rockefeller Foundation which also extensively supported German eugenicists(241, pg 20) and until the late 1930s, the Carnegie Foundation.(241)

These German eugenicists found a home in the Nazi Party which was also very attractive for young medical doctors after 1933, so much so that medical doctors constituted the largest professional group in the NSDAP (Nazi Party).(242)

This idea of improving the genetic stock led to the Nazi euthanasia program which was extensively supported by medical doctors(242) who were then easily recruited into medical research for biological warfare.

Why is this important? Much of medical research is expensive and needs to be financed. One of the biggest financers of medical research are sovereign governments who have an interest in healing their population but also have another strong interest in biological warfare which has substantial consequences for medical research.

During World War II medical doctors in Germany(243) tested the effect of bacteria and toxins on healthy subjects in order to be able to attack their enemy and vaccinate their own population or soldiers against those agents.

The Japanese went much further, with the Japanese Imperial Army Unit 731(24, 244) killing hundreds of thousands of people in Manchuria including vivisecting 3,000 people while alive without anaesthesia. The medical doctors performing these experiments were part of the Japanese medical elite and occupied many senior positions in Japan after World War II.(24) The reference here given is Robert F. Kennedy Jr's book 'The Wuhan Cover-up' which provides a large number of primary sources.

The United States was more interested in the medical knowledge gained by the German and Japanese medical doctors than in prosecuting them and used Operation Paperclip to bring a substantial number of these doctors over to the United States to engage in biological warfare and vaccine research.(243)

The United States kept up this biological warfare and vaccine research throughout with generous government funding including releasing biological agents on its own population for research purposes with much of the funding since 2000 being dispensed by Dr Anthony Fauci's National Institute of Allergy and Infectious Diseases (NIAID) including the gain-of-function research to make viruses more lethal, more infectious and easier to disperse.(24)

The Wuhan lab leak is likely only one of a number of laboratory leaks that led to disease outbreaks.(24, Chapter 27)

When there is a catastrophic failure of medical research then there is a strong motivation to cover up the cause of the new pathogen but in theory there are also vaccines available in short order as the vaccines were developed in parallel with the pathogen. A vaccine to inoculate a large part of the world population is a financial bonanza for pharmaceutical companies who keep the media onside through large spending on advertising and, if the vaccine is developed as part of gain-of-function research, those pharmaceutical companies also have strong political backing.

Once the scene for a seeming major crisis is set, the scientific method gets overridden in a public health emergency where it is more important to be seen to be doing something than whether the actions are scientifically or ethically sound, such as mandatory mask wearing,(55) social distancing, lockdowns, vaccine mandates and treatments for the newly emergent threat such as COVID-19.(53, 54) At the moment I cannot find scientific articles that outline the outrageous and unsound population restrictions that were instituted during the so-called pandemic, only links that show how people will go along with such coercive measures.(245, 246)

Within a few years from 2024 I expect that it is considered to be obvious that COVID-19, a gain-of-function enhanced coronavirus, spread from the Wuhan Institute of Virology in 2019 throughout the world. The Wuhan Institute of Virology has strong ties to the Chinese military and received substantial funding from Dr Fauci's Institute for gain-of-function research. Corona viruses are common and cause about 21% of common colds(247) and are different from the influenza virus(248) with this particular coronavirus having symptoms similar to influenza and a comparable death rate under normal circumstances,(39) with much depending on population health and treatments given.

Influenza epidemics are quite common, and a pulmonary (lung) specialist told me that those over 65 who are vulnerable and who get influenza have about a 20% mortality rate within 12 months, though influenza would rarely be noted as a cause of death. COVID-19 disproportionally affected those with chronic diseases and ailments such as diabetes and obesity and, as expected, those with suboptimal respiratory abilities and when it killed, it did so quickly, so even if the 12-months mortality would be the same as for influenza, many more deaths would be attributed to COVID-19.

From the moment that the alarm was raised for COVID-19 in late 2019 to early 2020, the scientific method was honoured in its breach by politicians and regulators taking measures for which there was no or contradictory scientific evidence. Importantly, most of those extreme and ubiquitous breaches were not flagged as such except by minority groups who were consistently vilified by the media. One prominent example, that actually was flagged, was the Lancet paper rejecting hydroxychloroquine as part of a COVID-19 treatment regime based on invented data,(249) leading to a very safe medication that can be given to pregnant women,(250) hydroxychloroquine (HCQ) being treated like this (FDA – United States Food and Drug Administration, HHS – United States Department of Health and Human Services):

> *"After widespread use of the drug for 65 years, without warning, FDA somehow felt the need to send out an alert on June 15, 2020 that HCQ is dangerous, and that it required a level of monitoring only available at hospitals. In a bit of twisted logic, Federal officials continued to encourage doctors to use the suddenly-dangerous drug without restriction for lupus, rheumatoid arthritis, Lyme and malaria. Just not for COVID. With the encouragement of Dr. Fauci and other HHS officials, many states simultaneously imposed restrictions on HCQ's use."(24, Chapter 1)*

The Lancet paper was retracted after extensive protests but the prohibition on hydroxychloroquine remained. The Lancet is one of the oldest and most prestigious scientific journals. Being published in The Lancet is a strong career boost for researchers.

Evidence-based medicine uses the scientific method and relies on the scientific method to be followed. If the scientific method is optional and guidelines can be created in violation of the results of the scientific method or if the scientific method is misused to provide authoritative misleading or outright false results, then evidence-based medicine is worse than any faith-based treatment method as we move from damage caused by individual practitioners to damage caused universally when evidence-based medicine makes sure that the best treatments are not available as has happened with ivermectin and hydroxychloroquine combined with zinc during the COVID-19 event.

As effective treatments were suppressed and ineffective measures such as many lockdowns(53, 54) and mask mandates(56, 251-253) together with ineffective or dangerous medicines(254, 255) were imposed, evidence-based medicine has been widely discredited and a much larger number of people became aware of extensive misuse of the scientific method and therefore the unreliability of the scientific method's declared results as shown in many of these citations and the studies the citations refer to. The long-term effects of this loss of respect may be substantial.

How to Use Research to Disseminate the Message You Want to Spread Regardless of the Facts.

If the remedy truly works though only when administered correctly and you need to prove that the remedy does not work – the below is a commonly used strategy.(60)

Hydroxychloroquine

Hydroxychloroquine is increasingly toxic when given in extra large doses and mainly or only works as a helper agent (ionophore) to let zinc, which is the active antiviral agent, enter cells infected with COVID-19. The reason that zinc needs a helper material is that zinc, due to its electrical properties cannot enter cells by itself(153, 256)

Therefore hydroxychloroquine is easy to discredit by overdosing, using it without zinc as hydroxychloroquine may or may not have antiviral properties by itself,(257) and using it on hospitalised patients as antiviral remedies work best when administered early.(258, "Early treatment is more effective")

This misuse was the employed configuration of the famous Recovery(259) and Solidarity(260) trials and similarly for a systematic review of 28 trials of hydroxychloroquine where the meta-analysis did not mention the word 'zinc'.(261) In addition, this systematic review gave 89% weight to the Recovery and Solidarity trials, making it almost inevitable that the systematic review had the same results as these two trials.(262)

Both trials involved huge logistics, setting up randomised controlled trials where patients were randomly assigned to either an experimental treatment or standard care, which in this case meant whatever the hospital used at the time for very sick COVID-19 patients. The hospitals were all over the world and the trials were conducted within months.

One part of the Recovery trial investigated whether hydroxychloroquine (HCQ) worked. In that trial, HCQ was given at only 23% less than a known toxic dose,(263) made worse by not considering the toxicity resulting from *"ignoring the very long half-life of HCQ and the dosing regimen - much higher levels of HCQ will be reached later."*(ibid.)(264)

Therefore, the Recovery trial used a medicine that works best when combined with the common supplement zinc in early stage COVID-19, without zinc, at a very late stage more than nine days after COVID-19 onset and only on the sickest as they were in hospital, with an increasingly incorrect toxic dose.

As a consequence, the Recovery trial had a death rate of 25% in the usual care arm and an even higher 27% in the hydroxychloroquine arm for an illness for which there was already, when the trial was run, multiple protocols available which combined HCQ with zinc. If the standard hospital care would not have been so ineffective at the time, then a death rate that is as high as 27% would have drawn a lot of attention.

Alternative treatment protocols for HCQ that included zinc were known as one of the proponents met President Trump after sending him a video on March 21, 2020(265) which was publicly referred to by President Trump and another famous researcher and medical doctor, Didier Raoult, met the French President Macron.(266)

Most people will remember Zelenko and Raoult as figures that were vilified by the media even though their proposed usage of HCQ as a COVID-19 treatment actually worked.(153)

As a consequence of the Recovery trial, an effective treatment was denied to millions of people while a lot of deaths happened in their trial. According to some, that is scientific misconduct on a grand scale and yet the protagonists were not held to any consequence, they were not affected in any public way and their official reputation remains intact.

These two trials then lead to one of the most highly cited researchers, John Ioannidis concluding that hydroxychloroquine does not work in a paper on hydroxychloroquine that also does not mention the essential zinc.(267)

A detailed timeline showing the information management about the effectiveness to hydroxychloroquine is given in these three fringe publications.(268-270)

When I speak to lay people about these trials that seemingly had been set up to fail, i.e. to show that a well-working medicine in the form of hydroxychloroquine was not working when it does work, such a concept of proving the opposite of the truth, makes sense to them as they regularly encounter rules and regulations whose sole purpose seems to be to make their work harder.

However, with medical researchers I have spoken to, this point about trials seemingly designed to fail, is more difficult to consider as in their experience the whole point of any medical trial is to make the world a better world by knowing more and finding out if a treatment works. The idea of knowingly designing a trial for a well-working medicine in such a way that the medicine does not seem to work is quite foreign and they look for alternative explanations.

Medical researchers understand trials, especially by pharmaceutical companies, that gild the lily, making the treatment look better and even make control treatments look worse(271) but to wholly pervert the idea of a medical trial and that at a worldwide scale with many thousands of people co-operating is from what I can see rarely part of a medical researcher's conceptual framework.

A temporal explanation could be that it was imperative that the world receives mRNA injections and for that the United States FDA's emergency use authorisation was needed which cannot be forthcoming if there are working treatments but that still leaves the question of why such wide-spread collaboration and why would these mRNA injections despite their side effects and their very limited if any reductions in infections or hospitalisations for COVID-19 be so important?

Why would researchers risk their professional careers and why would so many people co-operate and why would there not be an uproar eventually? That, and other facets of COVID-19 currently defy explanation and can only be described in factual detail until a true explanation is forthcoming. In the meantime, it is very useful to have a more open and less censored view of what is happening.

Playing both sides of the street: Professor John Ioannidis

COVID-19 exposed many enthusiastically practised perversions of medical research and also put established scientists and medical practitioners under pressure. John Ioannidis, also the author of the most downloaded research paper(142) before COVID-19, an essay titled "Why most published research findings are false" was famous for eloquently pointing out the shortcomings of medical research while being very much an insider as a Stanford University professor and receiving many honours as listed by himself in this essay on COVID-19 by him.(272)

During COVID-19 he authored early on in 2020 a WHO Bulletin(39) that showed that COVID-19's infection fatality rate was very low in many countries. This publication was very courageous as it was quite foreseeable that the publication would almost destroy his reputation as he received many attacks for supposedly downplaying the problem. By 2024 those findings were more or less accepted as accurate but that did not stop the firestorm of criticism in 2020 and 2021.

On the other hand, Professor John Ioannidis is a co-author in the previously mentioned systematic review that is a complete perversion of scientific medical research and it was clear at the time that that publication was an egregious misrepresentation of the effects of hydroxychloroquine.(261)

COVID-19 protocols widely circulating on the internet at the time pointed out that hydroxychloroquine needed to be taken with zinc to be effective and best early on, before hospitalisation.

Ivermectin

Ivermectin is a much more formidable opponent than hydroxychloroquine and works so well that those who work on discrediting ivermectin are discrediting themselves and are much more visibly exposing the way they pervert the scientific method. The discrediting of ivermectin is made harder by c19ivm.org, a website showing an ongoing, anonymous systematic review of 50+ COVID-19 treatments including ivermectin, as this website is run anonymously by experienced and highly published statisticians, judging from the level of expertise shown on the website.

When the project is to discredit ivermectin, having the media onside, which means your actions are not criticised, in fact supported by the media, is very helpful to such a discrediting project.(273)

The obvious beneficiaries of this manipulation, discrediting cheap at 10 cents per 12mg tablet, well-working antiviral treatments, were the vaccine companies, mostly Moderna, Pfizer and BioNTech as they earned billions and paid royalties of $710 million to NIH employees of which $690 million went to employees of the National Institute of Allergies and Infectious Diseases (NIAID) while Dr Fauci was director from 1984 to 2022(274) but for some reason the entire media bar some fringe publications and some 90% of all politicians and over 90% of health bureaucracies co-operated with this force even though many of the participants knew the true facts. It clearly was not just about the money as many administrators and politicians made themselves liable for future accusations of grievous bodily harm, murder and genocide without in many cases seemingly gaining any substantial personal advantage.

A commonly used tactic was to simply ignore the evidence on ivermectin and other remedies. That however, was not enough for medical researchers. Hence already published papers showing ivermectin's efficacy were retracted without good reason. (275) Therefore, research was produced that downplayed or discredited ivermectin and other remedies but there was also substantial research showing ivermectin's efficacy. The first line of defence was to only quote studies that showed no or little effect on COVID-19 by ivermectin and to simply ignore the overwhelming evidence provided by c19ivm.org.

The second line of defence uses a real problem, well expressed by John Ioannidis in his popular essay "Why most published research findings are false."(142) When there is a great deal of public interest in a particular research area, there are often or perhaps always people who cut corners in their research, providing partly or wholly fake results. The BBC used examples of fake or falsified studies that reported that ivermectin worked to tar all ivermectin studies except those that showed a negative result.(276)

One reason for the media being onside with the large pharmaceutical companies is because these companies provide a large part of their advertising income. In a Tucker Carlson interview (tuckercarlson.com) a statement was made that the pharmaceutical companies do not need the advertising exposure as they control the doctors (and the guidelines and the research) and advertise in order to influence the editorial cover of a media that is mostly desperate for funds.

This slanted coverage is damaging to any remaining credibility of the media which is losing customers in droves, leading to new owners who do not purchase newspaper, TV or other publishers to make a profit but for the new owners to have more power and political influence as it does not make financial sense to own chronic loss-making enterprises.

However, the ongoing reduction in audiences and aging of audiences(277), showing median ages of over 60 for United

States TV networks, leads to reduced influence, further reductions in headcounts and other costs, more dependency on advertisers and independently very wealthy owners, more unreliable coverage etc. until something changes, for example a media company being successful without habitually telling untruths.

The result is that any person who googles 'ivermectin' or uses Google Scholar will get a strong impression that ivermectin does not work as all the early Google hits and their listed studies show that ivermectin does not work or worse.

On a less slanted search engine, yandex.com, when searching 'ivermectin' with one exception(278) shows hits that cover its anti-parasitic effect and little about its effect on viral diseases including COVID-19. In March 2024, yandex.com on my searches showed c19ivm.org as the first hit when searching for 'ivermectin COVID-19'. All but the last hit on the first page of this second query's search results, which was Wikipedia expressing the view that ivermectin does not work, were to web pages that were positive on ivermectin. As all search engines take the user's previous searches into account, other people's results may differ substantially, however it has been well established that the media including Google paid a large hand in censorship and propaganda. They consistently made untrue and forceful statements, supporting the same purpose as those who considered it important that a large part of the world population receives mRNA injections rather than prophylactic measures and treatments.

Even now, in early 2024, the website c19ivm.org and its some 50 sister websites reviewing any researched COVID-19 treatment is almost completely unknown even in scientific circles. I showed the website to a number of post-docs and PhD students in mid 2023 during an online meeting where the subject was COVID-19 and the only person who commented chose to ignore the overwhelming evidence and evident quality of the website because one of the sister websites showed that hydroxychloroquine was an effective treatment and to them that was clearly wrong and therefore the entire set of websites could only be wrong. Nobody contradicted this assessment and the discussion was quickly shut down. It was quite remarkable to see that kind of so-called science in action.

If the Remedy Truly Works and You Need to Prove the Opposite to Scientists and the Sophisticated General Public.

The very large majority of people can be influenced through the media, whether legacy, social media or peer pressure. Many need not be convinced of the truth of your argument – here that vaccines work and existing antivirals do not work – but cower to threats to their employment or financial security if they speak up. Those that cowed included many doctors.

Then there are those with a scientific bent and medical researchers who for various reasons such as an income independent of medicine, retirement or imminent retirement and with the time to do research themselves that are harder to convince of outright and obvious lies. They need to be persuaded that black is white, that antivirals do not work and therefore all we have are vaccines as happened during COVID-19.

A successful such persuasion was by a popular general science blogger to marginalise proponents of ivermectin as a COVID-19 treatment. As shown, this is a formidable task as:

- the discoverer of ivermectin got the Nobel Prize for medicine for the discovery;(279)
- ivermectin is so safe that it can be given to pregnant women;(280)
- ivermectin is a very successful anti-parasitic of which the WHO gave out billions of doses in Africa;(281)
- it is successful in animal parasite treatments;(282)
- shows promise as a cancer treatment;(283-289)
- it can be used against all stages of COVID-19 from prophylactic to long COVID-19 where it has a strong, positive effect;
- and ivermectin is non-toxic even in large doses with few side effects.(290)

In other words, despite some expressed reservations, ivermectin is pretty much the ideal medicine.

As a curio, The Lancet is named after the tool used for blood-letting, a famously damaging therapy that was used for centuries until it was discredited.(117, 291)

One of the problems ivermectin has faced was that there was a strong global insistence and force for the entire world to receive mRNA injections(292-296) from 2021 onwards and that people were coerced into getting as many doses, called "booster shots" as possible.(297)

The injections could only be rolled out, ostensibly for COVID-19, if there was no existing remedy for COVID-19 because the FDA could then give an emergency authorisation for the injections to be approved(298, 299) and remove liability for the manufacturers(300) and governments could use coercive measures against those refusing the injections such as *"a) postponement or termination of the provision of social security or social assistance; b) suspension or termination of government administration services; or c) fines."*(292)

With ivermectin, the usual tactics of over- or under-dosing; administering too early or too late in the course of the ailment; quietly, without stating so in the trial reports, identifying those on the treatment and those on the control and treating them differently; etc., only worked to a limited degree as ivermectin is almost completely non-toxic (overdosing does not work), works in small quantities, not as well but enough to be identified as having a treatment effect through meta-analysis, works at any stage of COVID-19 and does not require any other treatment to show that ivermectin works. As ivermectin works while the virus is in the blood stream where it seemingly ties to one of two proteins the virus needs to enter cells but ivermectin has no effect on the virus while it is replicating in the cells, ivermectin is more effective in a full treatment regime but the problem for those who have to prove that ivermectin does not work is that that is not possible without drastic responses such as:

Running a trial in a location where ivermectin is freely available such as Colombia so the control group also routinely takes ivermectin. When both treatment and control group take ivermectin, it is difficult or impossible to show any difference in outcome between the groups. Another strategy is removing cases with a bad outcome from the treatment group or those with a good outcome from the control group, again reducing the difference in outcome, etc.

A trial that showed that ivermectin(301, 302) or hydroxychloroquine(259, 261) does not work then has a better chance to appear in one of the top journals. Each of these studies are heavily criticised here.(153, 238, 303)

However, there will, if there is sufficient interest such as during COVID-19, be too many trials that show that ivermectin works. Hence the next stage, which is to do a meta-analysis of all relevant trials to combine their results. In this meta-analysis one selects trials that favour the view that ivermectin does not work and rejects those that show that ivermectin does work.(304-307)

A very heavily substantiated example of this approach is written by what is most likely Dr Scott Siskind, a Californian psychiatrist in a popular blog "Astral Codex Ten", an anagram of his pen name Scott Alexander.(308, 309)

A Sophisticated Attempt to Discredit Ivermectin by Working a Meta-Analysis of Ivermectin Trials and the Response

Scott Alexander / Scott Siskind and his 19,000-word blog is countered by Alexandros Marinos (a true name) and his blog "Do Your Own Research" in a series of articles that encompass some 100,000 words. A 100,000 words is a common length for a full PhD thesis, while a book may have 40,000 – 60,000 words in many cases.(310)

The Astral blog's(308) strategy is to exclude a sufficient number of trials so that the meta-analysis becomes less powerful and individual trials more important. The effect of ivermectin then seemingly could be explained by a confounder, i.e. something separate that had an effect on COVID-19.

For this meta-analysis the theory was that ivermectin is also employed as an anti-parasitic in some regions and a person's parasitic load affects their COVID-19 response. The approach is faulty,(311, 312) summarised under both "*8. Reining it in*" and "*The Moral Argument*" in Marinos' paper but it is enough to convince many who kept looking for answers on ivermectin's effectiveness even after seeing the slanted Google searches and the biased Wikipedia entry.

The approach by Scott Alexander was successful in shaping opinions on ivermectin but does not work as a piece of scientific research as described, but that only became clear through the abovementioned detailed statistical analysis. For those interested in further details you can find a summary of that analysis here(311) and the greater details starting from here.(310)

More details on the meta-analysis

In order to discredit the meta-analysis of c19ivm.org(238) by providing an alternative meta-analysis, a chain of arguments needed to be created as mentioned before covered under "*8. Reining it in*".(311) Many scientists' first question when presenting a fact such as 'ivermectin works treating COVID-19' or 'ivermectin does not work treating COVID-19' is to ask for a systematic review or meta-analysis. The existence of c19ivm.

org's comprehensive meta-analysis then presents an incon-venience. Having an alternative meta-analysis, even if it is narrower and of inferior quality has the advantage of being able to provide a reply that suits those who want to state the opposite of the truth, the truth being that 'ivermectin works treating COVID-19'.

The first argument to use in creating an alternative, misleading meta-analysis is to reduce the number of studies by excluding all but early treatment studies. It is a commonly used method by making all investigated studies as similar as possible but one is then not trying to answer the question as to whether ivermectin works but whether it works as an early treatment. The purpose, though, is to reduce the number of studies, reduc-ing statistical power – the more studies, the clearer it becomes whether there is an effect or not. Reducing the number of stud-ies is a way to reduce the certainty of the effect.

The second step is to reduce the count of studies further by knocking out as many studies as possible as they may be biased, faulty, or fraudulent. If that does not work enough, one can use a method to establish which published papers have likely er-rors, a method that has a large rate of false positives (sound-ing the alarm when that is not justified), for example an often useful method by John Carlisle(313) which has a genuine good reputation but can be applied to create false alarms.

When that is not enough to get the desired result, step three is to cite a respected scientist who excluded further studies. Ignore evidence that this person is highly biased. Follow their example.

Then use a methodology that is not appropriate for this meta-analysis. You do not expect close scrutiny, so you use one of the simplest tests, which is a paired t-test where you still have a significant but by now borderline result (p=0.03), with the reduced number of studies.

However, because you have a small number of studies, you can look for other explanations that could explain away the now borderline result and you can then claim the conclusion you wanted to make.

In this case, the prevalence or not of a parasite was erroneously claimed to be a sufficient explanation for the treatment effect of COVID-19 to be explained by something other than ivermectin. A detailed analysis showed that that explanation did not work but such an analysis is rarely run on a respected figure's statement that quotes research published in the Journal of the American Medical Association (JAMA),(314) one of the top medical research journals.

That quoted JAMA published research took a different approach and therefore was not really compatible, but it serves the purpose of providing authority. A number of statistical measures were used, each of which can be sensible, but in aggregate were aggressive. Add in a 'serious flaw' to seemingly show that the ivermectin results were substantially different between countries where ivermectin was used as an anti-parasiticum vs countries where ivermectin was not used for that purpose when that difference is due to different scales used and that difference disappears when you use the same scale:

"As discussed in depth in my long-form article,(315) the second version contains a serious flaw which negates its statistical significance. While the paper says it is using only prevalence estimates from sources using parasitological methods (basically, stool sample examination), one of its two sources— used to obtain prevalence estimates for 10 of the 12 studies—in fact uses an adjusted blend of parasitological and serological methods (blood sample analysis). To demonstrate fairly intuitively, the estimates for the country of Brazil by the one source (Paula et al.)(316) is outside the 95% confidence interval of the other source's (Buonfrate et al.)(317) estimate for the same country. Therefore, this data cannot properly be used together without some adjustment.

When I did a fairly simple adjustment to line up the two data sources, the correlation in the dichotomous analysis weakened to the point of being even weaker than the original version (p=0.35), or as a frequentist [a statistician who prefers one of two major ways to interpret statistical results – the other type is called a Bayesian statistician (CS)] might say, 'there's no difference:'"

You can see how challenging it is and how much explaining is needed to follow a dispute when statistics are used. One reason is that statistics is not a settled science as shown in chapter 13(11) and can be used in many different ways to get many different results, though in this case Alexandros Marinos used methods that are very commonly accepted.

Here, Alexandros Marinos showed that even when the trial results of ivermectin are extensively manipulated, the evidence is still in favour of ivermectin as a working COVID-19 treatment.

Other Treatments of COVID-19

One of the benefits of discrediting existing, cheap and effective treatments when there is a large demand for a cure such as during COVID-19, is that there is a ready market for new treatments. Costs seem to matter little and research standards may be low.

Cost per life saved from NNT (Number Needed to Treat, a statistic that gives the number of people who need to take a particular remedy for one person to benefit. The higher the number, the less effective the treatment. Here NNT is used in conjunction with the cost of the remedy) in studies to day.

Treatment	Cost per life saved	Count of trials	Improve-ment
Melatonin	$8	9	48%
Vitamin D	$11	67	36%
Vitamin C	$14	39	19%
Zinc	$16	20	29%
Ivermectin	$24	51	49%
HCQ (Hydroxy-chloroquine)	$27	249	24%
Alkalinization	$28	5	42%
Vitamin A	$30	6	42%
Colchicine	$31	40	29%

Aspirin	$41	61	10%
Curcumin	$59	8	63%
Famotidine	$94	21	18%
Probiotics	$99	8	61%
Quercetin	$127	5	61%
Metformin	$155	60	34%
Antiandrogens	$175	33	38%
Nigella Sativa	$187	5	57%
Budesonide	$574	12	26%
Nitazoxanide	$680	6	42%
Azvudine	$1,237	12	35%
Fluvoxamine	$1,283	9	43%
Favipiravir	$1,717	38	12%
Tixagevimab/ cilgavimab	$74,506	10	42%
Molnuparivir	$137,653	17	23%
Regdanvimab	$139,860	3	70%
Casirivimab/ imdevimab	$181,694	8	40%
Paxlovid	$181,887	29	32%
Bamlanivimab/ etesivimab	$269,237	11	59%
Sotrovimab	$352,800	10	49%
Bebtelovimab	$737,601	4	60%
Remdesivir	$1,502,505	56	7%
Convalescent Plasma N/A	N/A	42	0%

Acetaminophen N/A	N/A	14	-24%
Source: c19early.org			

The interventions whose names end with 'vimab' seem to be monoclonal antibody treatments.

Molnuparivir is produced by Merck. Ivermectin was discovered by a Merck employee and sold by Merck while under patent. Merck published a statement(318) in 2021 on ivermectin:

> *"It is important to note that, to-date, our analysis has identified:*
>
> *- No scientific basis for a potential therapeutic effect against COVID-19 from pre-clinical studies;*
>
> *- No meaningful evidence for clinical activity or clinical efficacy in patients with COVID-19 disease, and;*
>
> *- A concerning lack of safety data in the majority of studies.*
>
> *We do not believe that the data available support the safety and efficacy of ivermectin beyond the doses and populations indicated in the regulatory agency-approved prescribing information."*

Comments by c19early.org/m on molnuparivir:

> *Potential risks include the creation of dangerous variants and mutagenicity, carcinogenicity, teratogenicity, and embryotoxicity. Multiple analyses have identified variants potentially created by molnuparivir. There is substantial publication bias. Multiple trials have not reported results and did not respond to requests. Molnuparivir has been officially adopted in 17 countries."*

Remdesivir from Gilead Sciences and Pfizer comments by c19early.org/s:

Remdesivir was used extensively in hospital for COVID-19 while excluding most other treatments.

> *"Studies show significantly increased risk of acute kidney injury. Remdesivir has been officially adopted in all or part of 37 countries. In November, 2020 only remdesivir and COVID-19 convalescent plasma were eligible for extra payments in the US from Centers for Medicare and Medicaid Services (CMS)."(319)*

c19early.org/p on paxlovid:

> *"Pfizer has denied access to Paxlovid for independent RCTs. Pfizer RCTs report very good results, while non-Pfizer RCTs show relatively poor results. Hoertel find that >50% of patients that died had a contraindication for Paxlovid. Retrospective studies that do not exclude contraindicated patients may significantly*

overestimate efficacy. Black box warning. The FDA notes that 'severe, life-threatening, and/or fatal adverse reactions due to drug interactions have been reported in patients treated with paxlovid'. Population studies often do not account for the different expected outcomes for the class of patients that seek out and receive early treatment. Paxlovid has been officially adopted in 35 countries."

c19early.org/ace on acetaminophen (paracetamol, a popular painkiller):

"Concerns have been raised over the use of acetaminophen (paracetamol) for COVID-19. Studies show significantly increased risk. Acetaminophen has been officially adopted in 44 countries."

No comments by c19early.org on convalescent plasma except that it has been officially adopted in one country (China).

As an example, as of early 2024, Australia adopted two monoclonal antibody therapies, acetaminophen (paracetamol), ibuprofen (a painkiller), paxlovid, remdesivir and budesonide. Only budesonide, a corticosteroid, at $574 to save one life is both reasonably successful and affordable.

It would be in keeping with the discreditation of effective, cheap antivirals that the commonly used, newly developed antivirals remdesivir and molnuparivir(154, 155) had little therapeutic effect as that kept up the seeming pressure to continue administering mRNA vaccines. It was also acceptable that remdesivir can cause substantial kidney damage.

In summary there were cheap, effective and harmless treatments and preventative medicines available from the start for COVID-19.

A large amount of money, media and governmental force was put into refuting these treatments, refuting the research and facts and instead insisting upon very expensive and harmful treatments. So called treatments that caused more harm than the condition they were purporting to treat.

COVID-19 Was Never Very Dangerous

The disease was not very dangerous in many countries even though each dominating slightly different version of COVID-19 quickly spread worldwide.

John Ioannidis caused a furore pointing the very low COVID-19 fatality rate early on(320) but later it became received wisdom. (321)

If the disease needs to be seen to affect many people

Seemingly Influenza almost disappeared during the COVID-19 epidemic(322-324) and there was no feared dual epidemic(325) with the physical effects of COVID-19 similar to the 2009 influenza epidemic.(326) Such a low rate of influenza incidences probably has not happened during recorded history. Influenza is and always has been quite dangerous for vulnerable people.(327-329)

COVID-19 was diagnosed via a PCR test, as outlined in Chapter 6, a test that would provide a false positive on many occasions, for example both COVID-19 and six viruses, that cause the common cold, are coronaviruses. The testers had strong financial motives to record a positive result, especially in hospital where subsidies were triggered on positive results.

Another misdirection was when people who died while testing positive in the recent past were often registered as a COVID-19 death, regardless of the actual cause.

COVID-19 is a disease that is usually only dangerous for older people who also have pre-existing co-morbidities and who in addition receive the wrong treatment as in no prophylaxis or early-stage treatment, the same people for whom influenza is a dangerous ailment.

This in population danger is equivalent to a severe flu or less, and yet was falsely broadcasted and branded as an epidemic and pandemic through selective and wide-spread media coverage, amplified by 'experts' with or without government authority and by politicians' pronouncements and enforced regulations and new legislation.

Preventing prophylaxis and treatment of COVID-19

It was known before 2020 that Vitamin D protects against respiratory diseases,(330) though this was put in doubt during COVID-19 in 2021(331) gaining the authors a publication in The Lancet, with a lesser publication confirming the benefit of Vitamin D in 2021(332) and another contradicting it in 2022.(333) It would make sense with the state of knowledge at 2020 during a respiratory epidemic to suggest Vitamin D supplements, exercise and sunshine as preventative measures to strengthen the immune system.

Instead the measures used were lockdowns,(53, 54) no treatment until a person became sick enough to require hospitalisation due to low oxygen levels, wearing masks indoors and outdoors, masks that make breathing harder, create a petri dish in front of your nose and mouth and do not reduce infections(55).

A measure not taken even though it is obvious and sensible for reducing the incidence and effect of respiratory illnesses was not to mention any supplements that strengthen the immune system such as Vitamins C and the abovementioned D. Even now, in 2024, there is no mention of such sensible prophylactic treatments.

Before 2020 there was a periodically updated Cochrane review on masks' influence on respiratory infections starting in 2006 and updated with no issue in 2007, 2010, 2011. This was updated again in 2020 and 2023 and became very controversial within the Cochrane foundation(334) including a Cochrane publication titled *"Policy makers must act on incomplete evidence in responding to COVID-19"*,(335) a seemingly uncontroversial statement except that the word *"must"* was used.

Masterful inaction as enacted by many poor countries, who should have been unusually vulnerable to a respiratory epidemic, worked far better than the actions taken in richer nations. The only action that 'worked' among richer countries were lockdowns in isolatable areas such as Australia and New Zealand but they came with a price that was completely out of proportion in damage to people's other health and wellbeing.

Examples of other harm included: fewer doctor visits leading to delayed diagnostics and treatments of other conditions, damage to population mental health including increased suicide and severe damage to the economy and exploding government debt, damage to small businesses with part of the destructive effects ameliorated by extensive government borrowing, essentially paying people not to work, thereby creating a sense of entitlement of getting paid for not working, and to pay businesses to be idle or work in a reduced capacity – a destructive cultural shift and dependency on government.

The measures taken are perfect to encourage uptake of vaccines, as people much prefer the ability to move around, but are highly detrimental to population health and finances.

The Testing Epidemic

During COVID-19 a very large number of people including asymptomatic ones got tested for COVID-19 using a polymerase chain reaction (PCR) test whose results were very unreliable. (158, 336) There are many pitfalls in using PCR tests as outlined in chapter 6 of this book.(157) The most extensively used manipulation was to increase the number of cycles – every cycle doubles the amount of genetic material that can be identified but also makes it more likely that a false diagnosis is made. Instead of the recommended 25 cycles, amplifying any material by a factor of 2^{25} = 33.5 million, 35 cycles amplifying by 34 billion or 40 cycles (1.1 trillion) were used.

A tool that should not be used for medical diagnostics was deliberately used in such a way that any viral material may have led to a false diagnosis, massively overstating the count of ill people. Hence the widely publicised concept of symptomless COVID-19. Add-in generous allowances and sick leave, creating an incentive to have a positive result and, especially in hospital, multiple tests until the result is 'right' and the COVID-19 government incentives will get paid. Furthermore, constantly publicise positive results and you can conjure up an epidemic where there is not one where hospitals had a strong financial incentive to overstate the supposed epidemic as COVID-19 patients attracted at least $175 billion in extra payments from the United States government through the CARES Act.(337)

Silencing Doctors

Doctors who protested COVID-19 measures were in danger of losing their license or did lose their license.(169, 171, 172, 338) A search for "losing medical license COVID-19" in Google gets lots of hits for justified licence loss due to misinformation and disinformation. On yandex.com it is more evenly divided. It wasn't until the end of 2024 that a suspended doctor had their license reinstated as the regulator did not state which law or regulation a doctor who protested against vaccines had violated.(339)

The terms misinformation and disinformation had a steady, lower, interest until 2020 and then substantially more interest with a different peak each in 2022 according to Google Trends. The terms are ill-defined and comprise both inaccurate and accurate but inconvenient information. The media uses them to imply false information but much accurate information, sometimes even from official government websites, is also labelled as misinformation or disinformation.

In summary, in this situation every aspect of evidence-based medicine was corrupted and that includes the reporting of false results while, when false results were asked for, those who provided accurate results were labelled as purveyors of misinformation or disinformation and sanctioned, including the abovementioned loss of license for doctors.

The reasoning, as explained here(172) is that it is deemed and insisted that vaccines work, therefore a doctor who expresses doubts about vaccines or proposes other treatments is engaging in misinformation or disinformation and therefore should not practise anymore, especially if the doctor is unrepentant.(171)

	Molnupiravir PANORAMIC Gbinigie, isrtcn.com	Ivermectin PRINCIPLE isrtcn.com(B)
Investigator	Prof. Chris Butler	Prof. Chris Butler
Delay	≤ 5 days from onset median 2 days	≤ 14 days from onset median unknown
Population	50+ or 18+ w/comorbidities	18+ (mid-trial change)
Treatment	5 days, 2x per day	3 days, 1x per day, dose below real-world use
Administration	Per recommendation (with or without food)	Directed to take opposite of recommendation for COVID-19 - without food, greatly reducing concentration cf 9ivm.org, Guzzo
Patients	25,783	est. 4,500
Publication delay	4 months	over 19 months (over 26 months from expected end), currently unreleased
Enrollment	Dec 2021 - Apr 2022	May 2021 - Jul 2022
Mutagenic	Yes	No
Cost	$707	<$1 medrxiv.org
Merck Profit	<$7.2B sales to date merck.com, estimated $18 to produce theintercept.com	~$0 (potential, unlikely competitive with low cost manufacturers)

Design better for showing efficacy

Design better for showing no efficacy

c19early.org

A Specific Example of a Heavily Manipulated Trial for Large Scale Information Management – The PRINCIPLE Trial of Multiple COVID-19 Treatments Including Ivermectin

"The PANORAMIC trial for molnuparivir and the PRINCIPLE trial for ivermectin provide a good example of extreme bias in trial design. For molnuparivir investigators randomized 25,000 patients a median of 2 days from onset.(238) For ivermectin, they allow inclusion up to 14 days after onset — a delay incompatible with the recommended use of antiviral treatments, and incompatible with current real-world protocols. This delay alone would normally be more than enough to guarantee a null effect for an early treatment. However, authors also bias the population, treatment dose and duration, treatment administration, and sample size to favor a null result with ivermectin."

The table and the comment below the table show how a medical trial can be extensively manipulated during the setup phase, making a positive result much more likely for molnuparivir and a negative result much more likely for ivermectin. As both trials were designed by the same person the difference in trial designs cannot be a coincidence and is clearly by design, showing just one aspect of how manifestly corrupt medical trials can be.

If research standards were important, a blatant tipping of the scales as above would end a research career, but this is not happening. It seems more likely that such measures are business as usual.(60) The above quote about the PANORAMIC and

PRINCIPLE trials was written before the release of the PRIN-CIPLE findings(276) where the abstract of the paper gives the required result:

> *"Ivermectin for COVID-19 is unlikely to provide clinically meaningful improvement in recovery, hospital admissions, or longer-term outcomes. Further trials of ivermectin for SARS-Cov-2 infection in vaccinated community populations appear unwarranted."*

Summary

In theory, there is a method that provides a workable way to get to the truth of what treatments in healthcare work and how well they work in the form of the medical research method.

In practice, the current manipulated way the medical research method is applied is associated with:

- no no increase in life expectancy;
- no the obesity epidemic;
- no a fake epidemic;
- no crimes against humanity through gain-of-function research;
- no a billion-person trial of unproven genetic therapy, excessive mortality in the 19-45 year olds(8, 215, 340, 341) with one of the four, a paper by Gibo at al, having been retracted against the wishes of the authors;
- no a now falling life expectancy for countries and subsets of populations;

- no a general deterioration in the health of children, including a very large rise in autism and auto-immune diseases;
- no a massive increase in treatments for mental health;
- no a substantial rise in the incidence rate of cancers, beyond what is expected of an ageing population and despite the benefit of widespread reductions in smoking;
- no global bankruptcy of healthcare systems and many more such harmful outcomes.

In other words, evidence-based medicine is wholly unsuccessful in reducing the incidence rates of illness and disease, including chronic and lifestyle diseases. It can be associated with better treatment of illness and disease but also with unsustainably rising healthcare costs.

It is hard to imagine a worse system for population health outcomes and misdirected costs. Evidence-based medicine in its application is associated with severe and ongoing damage to population health.

COVID-19 was an engineered boon for pharmaceutical companies with the extra support and contributory enforcement of the media, the regulator and the politicians but on the downside came unexpected levels of scrutiny of their practices from a large number of parties.

Biological warfare created a virus that leaked or was released in the wild and the response killed millions of people, impoverished nations, enriched pharmaceutical companies and vastly increased government powers.

CHAPTER 7

MUCH OF THE COVID-19 PLAYBOOK OF STRATEGIES HAS BEEN USED BEFORE AS PER PETER GØTZSCHE'S 2013 BOOK

There is nothing new under the sun – King Solomon, Ecclesiastes 1:9

Was this series of COVID-19-related events new or uniquely bad?

No, most strategies have been successfully used by pharmaceutical companies, their regulators and legislators for many years as Peter Gøtzsche's book from 2013 "Deadly medicines and organised crime"(60) describes in great detail.

Peter sets the scene with:

> "My book is not about the well-known benefits of drugs such as our great successes with treating infections, heart diseases, some cancers, and hormone deficiencies like type 1 diabetes. The book addresses a general system failure caused by widespread crime, corruption and impotent drug regulation".

He continues:

> "If you don't think the system is out of control, please email me and explain why drugs are the third leading cause of death in the part of the world that uses most drugs. [The United States] If such a hugely lethal epidemic had been caused by a new bacterium or a virus, or even one-hundredth of it, we would have done everything we could to get it under control."

In a new analysis in 2024, Peter Gøtzsche corrects this to prescription drugs being the leading cause of death and psychiatric drugs the third leading cause of death.(342)

Peter Gøtzsche's book is a detailed description of the corruption of "the best available evidence" by all participants in healthcare, pharmaceutical companies, regulators, doctors, and patients, and gives particulars on how evidence is manipulated so the declared "best available evidence" is not the "best" but the one that suits interested parties the most. It also shows how massive amounts of existing evidence are not "available" as the evidence is suppressed, ignored or discredited and how the evidence that is available is often false.

Therefore *"the best available evidence"* as provided in guidelines **is neither the best, nor available, nor evidence**.

One surprise for a reader of Peter Gøtzsche's book when it came out in 2013 would have been the amount of regulatory capture and corruption that was then already happening. The financial future of many senior employees of regulators depends critically on their future employment by pharmaceutical companies, an awareness that seems to have very much informed many regulators' actions.

A third highlight of the book is how many doctors allow corruption to flourish by the doctors acceding and not sufficiently complaining about corruption and how a minority of high earning, influential doctors are actively and knowingly acting against the interests of patients, in fact actively and knowingly harming many patients for personal gain. How far away is this behaviour from the Mengeles(343) and Shipmans(344, 345) of this world?

The Following Are All Interesting Quotes from Peter Gøtzsche's Book

From the foreword by Richard Smith, stating the book is making a case for these points:

> *"... the drug industry has systematically corrupted science to play up the benefits and play down the harms of their drugs." ... "the industry has bought doctors, academics, journals, professional and patient organisations, university departments,*

journalists, regulators, and politicians." … "very high proportions of doctors are beholden to the drug industry and that many are being paid six figure sums for advising companies or giving talks on their behalf."

From the foreword by Drummond Rennie:

"Gøtzsche's experience is unequaled. He has worked in sales for drug companies either as a drug company representative pitching pills to doctors or as a product manager. He is a physician and a medical researcher and has built a high reputation as head of The Nordic Cochrane Centre."

From the book:

"In the United States and Europe, drugs are the third leading cause of death after heart disease and cancer."

"The research literature on drugs is systematically distorted through trials with flawed designs and analyses, selective publication of trials and data, suppression of unwelcome results, and ghostwritten papers. Ghostwriters write manuscripts for hire without revealing their identity in the papers, which have influential doctors as 'authors', although they have contributed little or nothing to the manuscript."

Leading to:

> *"79% of US citizens said the drug industry was doing a good job in 1997, which fell to 21% in 2005,(346) an extraordinarily rapid decline in public trust.*
>
> *On this background, it seems somewhat contradictory that patients have great confidence in the medicines their doctors prescribe for them. But I am sure the reason patients trust their medicine is that they extrapolate the trust they have in their doctors into the medicines they prescribe. The patients don't realise that, although their doctors may know a lot about diseases and human physiology and psychology, they know very, very little about drugs that hasn't been carefully concocted and dressed up by the drug industry. Furthermore, they don't know that their doctors may have self-serving motives for choosing certain drugs for them, or that many of the crimes committed by the drug industry wouldn't be possible if doctors didn't contribute to them."*

Clinical trials explained through a third party quote:(347)

> *"WHAT IS A TRIAL? The approval process starts with evidence gleaned from clinical trials. It might be instructive to compare the sort of trials with which clinical researchers are familiar with those that go on in the courts. It seems to me fundamental that the legal trial carries credibility and retains force and respect with the public because the*

various parties, judge, jury, opposing counsels, witnesses and police, are independent one from another.

A clinical trial can be different. In that process, it is very much in the interest of the drug's sponsor, or manufacturer, to make everyone in the process its dependent, fostering as many conflicts of interest as possible. Before the approval process, the sponsor sets up the clinical trial – the drug selected, and the dose and route of administration of the comparison drug (or placebo). Since the trial is designed to have one outcome, is it surprising that the comparison drug may be hobbled – given in the wrong dose, by the wrong method? The sponsor pays those who collect the evidence, doctors, and nurses, so is it surprising that in a dozen ways they influence results? All the results flow in to the sponsor, who analyses the evidence, drops what is inconvenient, and keeps it all secret – even from the trial physicians. The manufacturer deals out to the FDA bits of evidence, and pays the FDA (the judge) to keep it secret. Panels (the jury), usually paid consultant fees by the sponsors, decide on FDA approval, often lobbied for by paid grass-roots patients organizations who pack the court (that trick is called 'astro-turfing'). If the trial, under these conditions, shows the drug works, the sponsors pay subcontractors to write up the research and impart whatever spin they may; they pay 'distinguished' academics to add their names as 'authors' to give the enterprise credibility, and often publish in journals dependent on the sponsors for their existence. If the drug seems no good or harmful, the trial is buried and everyone reminded of their confidentiality agreements. Unless the trial is set up in this way, the sponsor will refuse to back the trial, but even if it is set up as they wish, those same sponsors may suddenly walk away from it, leaving patients and their physicians high and dry.

In short, we have a system where defendant, developers of evidence, police, judge, jury, and even court reporters are all induced to arrive at one conclusion in favour of the new drug."

Misleading summaries of medical research:

"I have noticed on many occasions that these conclusions – and also often the results – in the abstracts of drug trials in the New England Journal of Medicine have been misleading. When I lecture doctors and tell them about this, I am usually met with hostile reactions. How dare I criticise the holy grail of medical journals, the very journal that all researchers hope to get into, if only once in a lifetime?"

Regulatory capture:

"When FDA scientists find signs of serious harms, they are often overruled and intimidated by their superiors – even to the point of being prevented from presenting their findings of lethal harms of drugs

at advisory meetings – or are assigned(348-350) to another job It doesn't even stop there. As described in Chapter 3, the FDA has accepted safety data it knew were fraudulent,(351) and – on many occasions – data that clearly showed the drug was not safe.(352)"

Quoting a former FDA scientist, Robert Kavanagh:(353)

"While I was at FDA, drug reviewers were clearly told not to question drug companies and that our job was to approve drugs ... If we asked questions that could delay or prevent a drug's approval – which of course was our job as drug reviewers – management would reprimand us, reassign us, hold secret meetings about us, and worse. ... Human studies are usually too short and the number of subjects in them too small to adequately characterize the most dangerous risks. That's why even a single case has to be taken seriously ...

if reviewers say things that companies don't like, they will complain about the reviewer or they will call upper management and have the reviewer removed or overruled. On one occasion, the company even told me they were going to call upper management to get a clear requirement for approval that they did not want to fulfill eliminated, which I then saw happen. On another occasion a company clearly stated in a meeting that they had 'paid for an approval' ... Sometimes we were literally instructed to only read a 100–150 page summary and to accept drug company claims without examining the actual data, which on multiple occasions I found directly contradicted the summary document. Other times I was ordered not to review certain sections of the submission, but invariably that's where the safety issues would be ...

FDA's response to most expected risks is to deny them and wait until there is irrefutable evidence postmarketing, and then simply add a watered down warning in the labeling ... When you do raise potential safety issues, the refrain that I heard repeatedly from upper management was, 'where are the dead bodies in the street?' Which I took to mean that we only do something if the press is making an issue of it ... Later, I found that the FDA had internal documents that had the same conclusion [as] my analysis but they had been withheld from the advisory committee ...

After FDA management learned I had gone to Congress about certain issues, I found my office had been entered and my computer physically tampered with. I saw strange cursor movements on my computer when I was just sitting at my desk reading that I suspected was evidence of spying ... The threats, however, can be much worse than prison. One manager threatened my children – who had just turned 4 and 7 years old – and in one large staff meeting, I was referred to as a 'saboteur.' Based on other things that happened and were said, I was afraid that I could be killed for talking to Congress and criminal investigators ...

I found evidence of insider trading of drug company stocks reflecting knowledge that likely only FDA management would have known. I believe I also have documentation of falsification of documents, fraud, perjury, and widespread racketeering, including witnesses tampering and witness retaliation"

Peter Gøtzsche on drugs being the third leading cause of death:

"Our drugs kill us on a horrific scale. This is unequivocal proof that we have created a system that is out of control. Good data are available,(354, 355) and what I have made out of the various studies is that around 100 000 people die each year in the United States because of the drugs they take even though they take them correctly. Another 100 000 die because of errors, such as too high dose or use of a drug despite contraindications. A carefully done Norwegian study found that 9% of those who died in hospital died directly because of the drugs they were given, and another 9% indirectly.(356) Since about one-third of deaths occur in hospitals, these percentages also correspond to about 200 000 Americans dying every year."

Polypharmacy, patients taking multiple drugs and the consequences:

"We know very little about polypharmacy

Most patients are in treatment with several drugs, particularly elderly patients. A Swedish study of 762 people living in nursing homes found that 67% were prescribed 10 or more drugs.(357) ... All these drugs may create cognitive impairment, confusion and falls, which carry a considerable mortality among the elderly. The symptoms are often misinterpreted by the patients and their carers as signs of old age or impending disease, e.g. dementia or Parkinson's, but when doctors stop the medicines, many of the patients apparently become many years younger, drop the wheeled walking frame, which they got because they couldn't keep the balance, and become active again. ... A randomised trial showed that drug reduction lowered both mortality and admission to hospital, and a subsequent study in 70 patients where number of drugs was reduced from 7.7 to 4.4 per patient showed that 88% reported global improvement in health and most had improvement in cognitive functions.(358)"

Corruption:

"It was very easy to corrupt doctors. Of 40 influential thought leaders identified as potential speakers in north-eastern United States, including 26 current or future department chairs, vice chairs, and directors of academic clinical programmes or divisions, no fewer than 35 participated in company-sponsored activities, and 14 requested or were allocated $10,250–$158,250 in honoraria or grants.(359) One doctor received almost $308,000 to tout Neurontin at conferences."(359)

Corruption helped along by pharmaceutical company:

> *"An internal [Pfizer] memorandum showed that doctors who attended dinners given by the company to discuss unapproved uses of Neurontin [only approved for treatment-resistant epilepsy] wrote 70% more prescriptions for the drug than those who didn't attend.(360) The company even insisted on pressing doctors to use much higher doses of Neurontin than those that had been approved, which means higher income for more harm.*
>
> *A seeding trial, the STEPS study, which had no control group, had the marketing objective to increase the dose of Neurontin and its market share, and it involved 772 physicians who only treated four patients each, on average.13 Physicians with little or no experience in trials were recruited and the data were very dirty, which the two published papers said nothing about. Drug salespeople collected data and were directly involved in suggesting to the doctors which patients to enrol while being present in the doctors' offices. The trial was deeply unethical, as the patients were not informed about the true marketing purpose of the study, and as the doctors were the actual study subjects without knowing this, as the effect of their participation on sales was closely monitored.*
>
> *Off-label promotion exposes patients to harms with no assurance of benefit. This criminal activity has increased and its victims have died, suffered heart*

attacks and strokes, had permanent nerve damage or lost their eyesight.(361) In 2010, a jury found that Pfizer violated the federal Racketeer Influenced and Corrupt Organizations Act (RICO) and the company was to pay $142 million in damages.(362) [2003 Neurontin sales were $2,700 million] The jury found Pfizer engaged in a racketeering conspiracy over a 10-year period."

Large scale deaths and injuries are normal for the FDA:

"Like Merck, the FDA failed badly in its duty towards the patients. A five times increase in heart attacks in the millions of people taking the drug [Vioxx] wasn't a public health(363, 364) emergency in the FDA's eyes. ... More than 80 million patients have been treated with rofecoxib [Vioxx],(365) and since about 10% of such events are fatal, a crude estimate is that rofecoxib has killed about 120,000 people."

Regulatory corruption:

"Pfizer has provided a most bizarre example of me-again. Aricept (donepezil) was the biggest player in the lucrative market for Alzheimer's disease with over $2 billion in annual sales in the United States alone.(366) Four months before the expiry of the patent, the FDA approved a new dose, donepezil 23mg, which would be patent protected for three more years, whereas the old doses of 5 and 10mg were not. The advertising was directed towards patients and contained untrue statements, but the scam worked."

"One would have hoped people were clever enough to take either 20 or 25mg of the drug to save money, but no. And the FDA failed us badly again. Its own medical reviewers and statisticians recommended against approval, as the 23mg dose didn't produce a clinically meaningful benefit whereas it caused significantly more adverse events, particularly protracted vomiting. The reviewers added that the adverse events could lead to pneumonia, massive gastrointestinal bleeding, oesophageal rupture and death.(367) This didn't impress the director of the FDA's neurology division, Russel Katz, who overruled his scientists."

Diagnosing:

"With such an approach to diagnosis [labelling normal behaviour as signs of depression], it's easier to understand why the rate of depression in the population has increased a thousandfold [to 9% of the US population] since the days when we didn't have antidepressant drugs.(368) ... when therapists have been asked to use DSM criteria, a quarter of healthy people also get a psychiatric diagnosis."(369)

Psychotropic drugs work, though not in the way expected:

"Psychotropic drugs don't fix a chemical imbalance, they cause it, which is why it is so difficult to come off the drugs again. If taken for more than a few weeks, these drugs create the disease they were intended to cure.(368, 370) ...

People may get terrible symptoms when they try to stop, both symptoms that resemble the disease and many others they have never experienced before. It is most unfortunate that almost all psychiatrists – and the patients themselves – interpret this as a sign that they still need the drug. They usually don't. They have become dependent, just like a junkie is dependent on heroin or cocaine, and as ADHD drugs and SSRIs [a widely used type of anti-depressant] have amphetamine effects, we should view these drugs as narcotics on prescription and use them as little as possible."

Bad consequences:

"The companies claimed that only 5% of the patients [using SSRIs, antidepressants] were sexually disturbed,(368) which is one-tenth of the true occurrence. In a study designed to look at this problem, sexual disturbances developed in 59% of 1022 patients who all had a normal sex life before they started using an antidepressant."(371)

Summary

In 2013 the media and politicians were easily manipulable and in most cases did little to improve affairs for patients. The regulators were captured to a substantial degree by product providers, and patients did not act against the systematic abuse on their bodies. By the time COVID-19 came along, the media, regulators and politicians and thereby the large majority of the public switched to actively supporting the agenda of 'vaccinating' the entirely population against overwhelming evidence that this was not needed and was in fact very harmful as outlined elsewhere in this book.

There is currently no good explanation for the worldwide uniformity among the media's lock-step output and the harmful healthcare related political decisions that are made in unison in many countries. A possible explanation for the United States is that pharmaceutical companies' advertising makes up a large proportion of most media organisations' budget but that is not the case in many other countries that employed exactly the same damaging COVID-19 related measures, often even more intensely.

COVID-19 provided an opportunity for pharmaceutical companies to make very substantial profits at the cost of the lives and injuries of millions of people, but pharmaceutical companies have made substantial profits at the cost of the lives and injuries of millions of people for a long time. The only difference is that more people noticed in this instance but most of those who noticed during COVID-19 are still unaware of all the other areas in healthcare where exactly the same pattern is repeated.

What happened with COVID-19, in particular was a widespread panic over a virus that, unless major errors in its treatment were committed, was no worse than influenza in its lethality.

This panic which was in stark contrast to the initially complete and over time almost complete indifference to the deaths and disablements caused by the newly developed drugs and vaccines to treat COVID-19, is what has been happening for decades and really for centuries with for example many centuries of bloodletting(291) and not using aether or ether(372) despite its known anaesthetic properties for surgery until 1846(373) when it had been known for centuries at least since 1540.(374, 375)

CHAPTER 8

WHY IS IT POSSIBLE FOR EVIDENCE-BASED MEDICINE TO CONTROL MEDICAL DOCTORS?

Historical Context

Up until the 1980s there was little oversight of doctors. As a consequence, many doctors abused their privileges by performing unnecessary procedures, charging too much, not learning from their mistakes and not taking advantages of the substantial opportunities to improve their work such as using more efficient processes that do not interfere with the quality of care.(63)

The quality of patient outcome and at what cost varied massively between practitioners and between regions.(63, 376)

"Many doctors had barely earned a middle-class living in the 1950s."(377) as medical doctors could not make much difference to a person's health up until the 1920s but in the next decades could treat diabetes with insulin, treat anaemia, treat infections with antibiotics, treat infectious diseases, and, with the help of better sanitation many diseases such as tuberculosis, typhoid, dysentery and the death rate from childhood diseases dropped dramatically.(63) It took 50 years from the 1920s for doctors' incomes to reflect these improved outcomes but it happened by the 1970s. It also meant that house calls by doctors became scarcer during the 1970s and onwards.

Due to the elimination of many childhood deaths, the benefits of sanitation and likely due to better medical care, life expectancy improved substantially during that period.

It also meant that as doctors got paid more without being more efficient in the management of their caseload, costs soared exponentially as demand increased with there being more and more treatments that were effective when needed. This was exacerbated in the United States by permissive legislation that made much more government money available. In the United States(378) over 60% of all medical expenses are covered by government at various levels. Further, the fact that much health insurance was paid by employers and not individuals, individuals seemingly had little incentive to control costs.

A particularly stupid legislative move in the United States, among many, was that health insurance companies could only make a profit of up to 20% of turnover(379, 380) or, more precisely, had to pay out 80% or more of turnover for healthcare costs: The consequence of that was that insurance companies had no interest in cost control as higher healthcare costs meant higher profits for them.

Doctors Losing Control

No oversight and a lot of money led to the predictable abuses of over-servicing, unjustified charging and substantial inefficiency. Over time during the 1980s and 1990s there were more and more initiatives, mostly from companies facing soaring health insurance bills, to reduce costs and later improve efficiency. This was helped along by legislation that forced companies to account for future healthcare costs on their balance sheet, increasing the incentive to have more efficient healthcare.(63)

Any attempt at reducing costs or improving efficiency was met with vehement protests by hospitals and medical doctors who thereby lost credibility as they did not provide their own oversight and showed, as a group, no interest in improving the efficiency of healthcare.

The massive increase in costs meant that those who directly paid for healthcare in the United States, mostly companies and governments, put more and more conditions on the money spent on healthcare. As doctors and hospitals did not participate as equal partners in these initiatives, they were sidelined from the decision process.

The main tools used for control were managing the minutia of healthcare through Health Maintenance Organisations (HMOs) and, from the mid 1990s, evidence-based medicine.

As doctors lost control to external entities, the entities that used evidence-based medicine as their lever could take control.

Depending on the type of call by the people, who are the ultimate enablers, doctors were controlled through different structures. In the United States it was an emphasis on maximising the amount of healthcare on offer and the more sophisticated the better. This turned out to be a toxic mixture of paying more per person on healthcare than any other country and having worse outcome than most developed nations, as medical care and an emphasis on specialist rather than primary care past a certain level is actually detrimental to population health.(131, 132, 205)

Other countries used different measures to control costs, such as a single government provider like the UK's NHS with little private (client paid) healthcare or the Australian Medicare system with a larger privately paid component. All of the systems control doctors to varying levels and this control allows decisions that are neither in the interests of doctors or patients even though they are those who are in one of the best positions to evaluate the usefulness of healthcare measures. Medical doctors have mostly dealt themselves out of the loop.

The above is well documented with copious examples in Michael Millenson's book "Demanding medical excellence: Doctors and accountability in the information age".(63)

Interesting Quotes below from Michael Millenson's Book "Demanding Medical Excellence: Doctors and Accountability in the Information Age" With Comments:

> *"why have forty years of scholarly studies and intermittent public scandals failed to make a significant impact [on health care costs]?"*

> *"Can the death toll from medical mistakes really be reduced? There's compelling evidence in the real world that a radical reduction awaits only the willpower to make it happen."*

The willpower has since been applied but the remedy was centralisation leading to widespread corruption and deaths came about in different ways such as iatrogenic treatments where the treatment is harmful. Obvious examples are over-diagnosis, false positives in tests and the many issues with pharmaceuticals.

> *"In submitting evidence to satisfy these rules, drugmakers were required by law to produce data collected from "adequate and well-controlled investigations, including clinical investigations." FDA guidelines emphasized that no drug would be approved unless it underwent a clinical trial whose protocol was approved by the FDA and whose results were reviewed by the agency and critiqued for accuracy and completeness. Objective evidence had dealt empiricism a resounding defeat."*

How did empiricism strike back? By offering FDA employees secure, highly paid jobs after their stints.

> *"Continuous quality improvement took the structure more or less for granted, honed in on every step of process, then measured the resulting alteration in outcome."*

The problem in United States medicine is in large part the structure with too many specialists, disempowered GPs or family physicians, pharmaceutical companies that are too powerful and therefore captured regulators and legislators.(139) This is enabled by the public who works on the assumption that more medical care and more pharmaceuticals are better plus a myriad of consequences due to this set of expectations.

> *"The individual physician's near-unlimited authority to interpret the medical literature was being replaced with a group interpretation. Doctors had to trust their colleagues who drafted the guidelines, even if they did not know those colleagues personally. This leap of faith was tough enough when treatment of one clinical condition (pneumonia, heart attacks, tetralogy of Fallot) was at issue. It was even more difficult during a disruptive period when doctors were being told to standardize virtually their entire practice. To reassure doctors that standardization was not a weapon for forcing them into "cookbook medicine," ICSI adopted the rule used by Salt Lake City's LDS Hospital: **if a doctor disregarded a guideline, the doctor was presumed right and the guideline**

wrong until it was shown otherwise. The final change in medical practice".

Evidence-based medicine reversed this onus. Today, if the doctor disregards a guideline they may and often do have to substantiate their decision to the regulator or in a medical tribunal or court case. This gives too much power to guidelines and therefore to those who write the guidelines and therefore to those who can support, influence or corrupt the authors of guidelines and those who appoint the authors of guidelines and those who appoint the appointors of authors of guidelines, none of whom seem to have much if any accountability for their choices themselves.

History of Medicine for the Last Century

"By the beginning of the twentieth century, biomedical research began yielding the kind of tangible benefits that the physical sciences had begun to contribute years before. In the 1920s came the discovery of insulin as a treatment for diabetes mellitus and the use of liver as a cure for anemia, which until that time was fatal. By the mid-1930s, physicians could prescribe a few tablets of the new sulfanilamide drugs to vanquish infectious diseases that used to devastate entire communities.(381) The death rates for tuberculosis, typhoid fever, meningitis, measles, dysentery, and whooping cough plunged between 1900 and 1935 owing to a combination of better medical care and long overdue improvements in public health and sanitation.(382)"

"Reflecting this public faith in medical science, federal funding for biomedical research exploded twenty-five-fold in a decade, jumping from less than $3 million in 1941 to an astonishing $75 million.(383) Until the 1980s, the growth remained exponential. (384)"

"Many doctors had barely earned a middle-class living in the 1950s."

"By the late 1960s, about 90 percent of the United States population had private or public health insurance that reimbursed on a fee for service basis just about any care doctors and hospitals deemed necessary. This did not, however, lead to a period of national good health and good cheer. Instead, it was a time of unprecedented anger and dissatisfaction with American medicine. The epidemic of unneeded surgeries and the growing number of treatment-related injuries and deaths had finally led to widespread public outrage. Public disillusionment with unfettered physician autonomy was so complete that Congress came very close to passing national health insurance."

If you can write your own check, it tends to be big. If you abuse your mandate without controlling the media and you abuse your mandate to such a degree that the media publishes reports of widespread anger, then you allow others to control you.

"... uncontrolled greed in medicine is what enabled managed care to take power in the first place." And

"Prospective payment provided two critical insights into cost control. First, it showed that substantial waste could be eliminated without harming patient care, even if community physicians and hospitals complained bitterly all the while."

When the public flexes its muscles through a compliant media:

"It was by any measure an unusual scene. Hospitals that had always focused on making themselves attractive to doctors were forced by the marketplace to invest millions of dollars to make themselves attractive to patients."

"Surgical anesthesia was first publicly demonstrated on 16 October 1848 at the Massachusetts General Hospital. John Collins Warren's removal of a jaw tumor from Gilbert Abbott under the influence of William Thomas Green Morton's Letheon sent shock waves around the world. By the end of the year, Europe was experimenting with this new American discovery. Yet, at the turn of the nineteenth century the anesthetic properties of nitrous oxide had been discovered by Humphry Davey working at the Bristol Pneumatic Institute. Why did it take almost a half century from the initial observations of insensibility to surgically induced pain, to the application of anesthesia?"(374)

"Emanuel Papper, a world-renowned anesthesiologist, wrote that the ability of ether to dull pain was known for centuries before anyone thought of applying it to making surgery less agonizing. Suffering was

> *associated with nobility of spirit or viewed as a*
> *punishment for sin. "It took so long to discover*
> *'anesthesia,'" wrote Papper, "because there was no*
> *societal readiness for it nor interest in the prevention*
> *of the pain of surgical intervention or really in the*
> *relief of pain for the common man."(374)*

It is quite possible that anaesthetics were used informally on a small scale beforehand, but I was quite surprised at the obvious not being used for centuries. I find Pepper's explanation not convincing but do not have a better explanation.

> *"As one JAMA [a top medical journal] commentary*
> *put it in early 1997: "The dream of medicine for the*
> *new millennium [is] that the care of patients will*
> *be evidence based, supported by carefully designed*
> *randomized controlled trials and validated by*
> *focused outcomes studies."*

The dream has come true, and it is a nightmare as the trials and studies, their reporting and the implementation of their findings have been corrupted.

> *"In fiscal 1997 the National Institutes of Health*
> *received $12.7 billion [$51 billion in 2024]; AHCPR*
> *[now AHRQ] got $143 million [$564 million in*
> *2024], or about one-hundredth as much."(385) ...*
> *"Systematic measurement and improvement of*
> *everyday medical care [the remit of AHRQ] may not*
> *be as glamorous as searching for the next 'magic*
> *bullet,' but it can save tens of thousands of lives*
> *right now if we help."*

The budget for improving the quality of care for which AHRQ is responsible is still only 1% of the budget for healthcare research even though it is obvious that improving the quality of care would improve millions of people's treatment experience. This missing the obvious is a parallel to not using anaesthetics for surgery for centuries and possibly millennia.

CHAPTER 9

THE INITIAL ELATION FOLLOWED BY THE LET-DOWN OF EVIDENCE-BASED MEDICINE

Many Times Evidence-based Medicine Is Superior to Doctors' Judgments

There are many examples of conventional medical wisdom before the rise of evidence-based medicine causing great harm to patients, from radical mastectomies being no better in their patient survival rates in the years after surgery than total mastectomies(134) to those, mentioned in Michael Lewis' bestseller, *The Undoing Project*, a book which is about Daniel Kahnemann and Amos Tversky showing the systematic fallibility of both lay and expert opinion.(386) Also evidence-based medicine is responsible for better heart attack and stroke care and other remedies.(17, 115-117, 134)

An example given in the Michael Lewis book was that it was conventional wisdom to suppress arrhythmia in patients after heart attacks, but evidence-based research showed that this increased rather than decreased mortality.

There are many such examples, but the same book also gives an example where intuition or a physician's judgment saved a patient's life as the initial diagnosis was wrong and treatment on that basis would have killed the patient.

Michael Lewis' book lists many examples and research that shows that human judgment is systematically flawed and that there are many cases where evidence-based medicine clearly improves the outcome compared to using a doctor's opinion.

However ...

Many Times Evidence-based Medicine Is Not Superior to Doctors' Judgments

The big subject of Michael Lewis' book(386) is that you can strongly influence lay and expert perception, opinion and understanding through framing. People will draw different conclusions if you frame a situation as one of choosing between different gains than if you frame the same situation as one of choosing between different losses, as people value avoiding losses higher than making gains. How do you frame the same situation as either choosing between gains or between losses? In the first case you ask people to choose between, for example, a gain of $1,000 or they will receive $2,000 and will lose $1,000. It is the same situation, but it feels quite different to the recipient.

This framing applies in many other cases, and I wonder if much of the convincing evidence for the superiority of evidence-based medicine is also a case of framing.

Just as it is possible to construct or narrate many real-life scenarios showing the evident superiority of evidence-based medicine over *"good old boys sat around a table"*,(119) would it be equally possible to frame a lot of scenarios that show a clear superiority of doctors' judgments?

Obvious examples are treating multi-symptomatic patients, patients who are on multiple drugs, scenarios where evidence-based research is ambiguous, or the guidelines are plain wrong. The many cases where the gathering and dissemination of evidence-based medicine has been corrupted, often systematically so with medical trials whose results cannot be replicated or that were manipulated for a stakeholder's outcome, bias through corruption or carelessness by medical publishers and their unpaid reviewers, misjudgement by a regulator and corruption in the production of guidelines. All these damaging activities happen in parallel to non-corrupt versions of these same activities and it may be postulated that the more money is at stake, the higher the incentives are to act corruptly.

Therefore, a doctor's judgment could also be superior where evidence-based research has been corrupted. Equally, a doctor's judgment could also be corrupted due to accepting financial favours or surrendering to regulatory force or a lack of time or interest to do their own research.

Would it need both evidence-based research and clinical judgment? If both are corrupted, no. The big difference between corrupted evidence-based medicine and corrupted doctors' judgment is that the former causes population-wide or even worldwide harm, the latter only causes individual harm. What is needed is for doctors to be liberated from the burden of proof when they do not adhere to guidelines. Such a measure will lead to much individual harm as doctors are fallible but also to many individual patients' benefit for the many cases where the guidelines are harmful due to corruption or non-applicability such as for patients who use multiple interventions.

Such a state of affairs may also motivate both doctors to step up as they can provide and publish successful case studies more easily, not having to fear sanctions for being at variance to guidelines and such a state of affairs may motivate guideline writers to improve the quality and integrity of their output as low-quality guidelines are more likely to be ignored.

Thus the question whether both evidence-based research and clinical judgment question are needed sounds trivial but in practice the current dominance of evidence-based medicine (for example *"In the UK National Health Service, all doctors, nurses, pharmacists and other health professions now have a contractual duty to provide clinical care based on best available research evidence"*,(119 5th edtn, pg 138)) but in practice, due to the dominance of evidence-based medicine, medicine in general as practised today, seems to be less and less interested in clinical judgment and more and more following and enforcing prescriptive rules.

For many medical practitioners these requirements could be quite demoralising if and when the guidelines go against their intuition or experience or when the guidelines are plain wrong.

Hence, it is quite possible that doctors who emphasise evidence-based medicine could have significantly poorer outcomes for a proportion of their patients than doctors who use their intuition and their own heuristics (judgment based on experience) as well. The opposite could also be the case, but for the moment the irony is that there is no evidence that the current high level of emphasis on using evidence-based medicine leads to better outcomes, except in the specific cases where there is clear evidence that traditional practices developed through expert consensus are inferior to evidence-based practices.

There are many anecdotes such as an often observed improvement in residential aged care patients (patients who need 24 hour medical resources on site) who had their copious medication removed with only necessary pharmaceuticals reintroduced together with a small amount of research in the matter. (387, 388)

One interesting outplay of evidence-based medicine is an oft-cited 2003 study from the RAND institute which says that most patients do not receive enough care, ranging from 79% of recommended care to as little as 23% for hip fracture and 11% for alcohol dependence.(389) An issue that arises about this study is that the data was collected under the assumption that the judgment of a person reviewing medical records only is equal or superior to the judgment of a doctor meeting the patient. The doctor meeting the patient may have good reason not to engage in all recommended medical practices and, in addition, there may be a wide range in the quality of the recommendations which means that many doctors may have good reasons not to agree with some, many or all of the recommendations.

Even if, after considering the above, there is still widespread underutilisation of recommended practices, it may simply reflect constrained finances, and this may not necessarily be to the detriment of the patients. Some patients will lose out on necessary care while others may benefit from, for example, not encountering false positives and the resulting wild goose chase for a medical condition that does not exist.

Hence, the oft-cited conclusions from the RAND study could easily be completely wrong.

It seems so obvious that evidence-based practice is better than the prior, clinical based judgment model that it simply is not publicly questioned whether evidence-based medicine is the superior approach and hence there is no research to consider whether evidence-based medicine as practised today is in fact a better approach on a population wide level than the current guidelines-based approach. Any deficiencies in evidence-based medicine should be improved through more or better evidence-based medicine is the prevailing paradigm.

Clearly this is a paradoxical question – using evidence to question the value of using evidence. But if we limit our acceptance of what we consider to be truthful to a single tool (scientific evidence), then we are stuck with it for as long as we hold that opinion. The research method is neutral. It can be used to support population health or it can be used corruptly. Where evidence-based medicine replaces flawed judgments, it has been successful.

We are back at the beginning – when we replace a search for truth with a set of prescriptive rules, we eliminate a lot of bad judgments, judgments that people in power claimed as their pronouncements of the truth. We allow those who are able to follow these rules – academics and businesses who run medical trials and providers of drugs and medical devices and a large bureaucracy – to control who gets what treatments, to control the process of accepting treatments and the experience and intuition of clinicians is de-emphasised in medical training and in practice through the emphasis on evidence-based medicine.

The rules and prescriptions of evidence-based medicine break down where patients have multiple ailments, a condition that is getting more and more prevalent with an ageing population, as the evidence of research results itself is flawed or deeply flawed(142); where clinicians are overwhelmed by the volume of the evidence and also de-motivated by the frequent changes, as new evidence is being presented that often contradicts previous evidence.

The premise of evidence-based medicine is that there is a benefit in replacing the intuition and experience of clinicians with evidence-based practices and procedures.

That may be true in individual cases but the disadvantages of this approach are widespread exhaustion or burnout which is defined as depression at work but not outside work(175, 390, 391) among medical practitioners and a population that is getting sicker despite a sharp increase in the cost of healthcare.

One approach is to try to make evidence-based medicine more patient centric(120), a call that has received a big response as evidence-based medicine may be intrinsically unable to allow a patient-centric model and thus, both strands of medicine need to be pursued separately at present. The call has received refutations(392) including one from the very prestigious British Medical Journal's (BMJ) editor-in-chief.(393)

CHAPTER 10

HOW DOES EVIDENCE-BASED MEDICINE GATHER ITS EVIDENCE?

Introduction

This is a big subject, but in outline there is a series of procedures at the end of which a practice or a tool will be accepted as either having sufficient evidence or not.

A good example is a new potential cancer remedy.

For instance, a particular chemical compound attacks cancer cells in the laboratory.

This compound then gets tested on animals, typically mice or rats. If it seems sufficiently safe, the compound then gets tested on a small number of humans to see whether it is also sufficiently safe for humans and what dose is (still) safe. This is called a Phase I trial.

If there is a safe dose, a slightly larger group of people is tested to see if the compound works, a Phase II trial. The next step, Phase III, is expensive, typically a double or triple blind randomised controlled trial where the compound gets tested against a placebo or the available standard treatment to see how well it works. Double blind means neither the doctor nor the patient knows which treatment has been administered. Triple blind means the person evaluating the data does not know which is which either – they just check if there is a difference between the two treatment methods or compounds.

If the compound passes all these tests, the developer can then sell the drug under patent protection until the patent runs out. Once the patent protection runs out, other companies can also sell that compound as a generic medicine, typically at a substantially lower price.

What Can Go Wrong In This Medical Research Process?

An enormous number of factors. The news is full of examples where the process has gone wrong.

For example, from a 2014 Scientific American article(394) it costs $1.4 billion to develop a new drug plus $1.2 billion in the fact that the money is spent over 10 years and could not be put to other use. This is an industry number and almost certainly exaggerated as Peter Gøtzsche estimates the amount to be closer to $100 million,(60) but even a number that is only one tenth of the $1.4 billion will mean that most promising compounds might never be investigated. In view of such high costs, only drugs that can sell well will ever be considered or drugs, such as vaccines, where the provider has limited or no liability, which leads to its own problems.

Hence, we now have drugs like the successful hepatitis C remedy(395, 396) that cost $70,000 or more per treatment and we may be running out of antibiotics as the market for a new antibiotics is often too small to pay for the development costs.

Every step of this procedure is full of errors and weaknesses.

Here is a small selection of them:

The first step in the above process is finding out whether a compound does what it should in the laboratory. In a well-known study,(397) Bayer Health Care revealed that in about two thirds of all cases, research findings cannot be reproduced. The drug companies are the victims here as they have been given false information and then spend a lot of time and money to see whether things really work – they are caught by the fact that most published research findings are false.(142, 398)

As far as the animal testing phase, apart from the ethical issues, animals are different from us. Penicillin is lethal for hamsters(399) and would not pass animal testing regulations today. Other differences mean that compounds either work better or worse in humans. In the latter case, the compound will not get past the animal testing stage, even though it should.

The human test phases can be endlessly manipulated, both to make a compound look better or worse than it is.

Why would a company make a compound look worse? When a drug comes out of patent protection, the drop in profits for the producer is usually large, as they lose their monopoly. One tactic that is reported to have been employed in some cases is to have a very similar replacement drug ready with a new period of patent protection,(400) a process called evergreening, and to publish a study that shows the old medicine in a bad light, which means the old medicine will have to be withdrawn from the market.

For the pain killer OxyContin, near the expiry of the original patent, the owner of the patent brought out a newly patented, seemingly safer version of the drug. As a consequence, the sale of the older version and its generic competitors was disallowed in many United States states, providing further monopoly profits to the producer of OxyContin.(401)

Another example is from Peter Gøtzsche(60) where regulatory capture allowed Pfizer to get a new patent for 23mg of the biggest Alzheimer's drug aricept (donepezil) after the patents on 5mg and 10mg ran out, increasing profits and side effects and neither doctors or patients figured out that they could simply prescribe 20mg or 25mg, if that was indicated, using multiple now-unpatented pills.

> "The [FDA] reviewers added that the adverse events could lead to pneumonia, massive gastrointestinal bleeding, oesophageal rupture and death.(367) This didn't impress the director of the FDA's neurology division, Russel Katz, who overruled his scientists."

The many ways to make a drug look better than it is, are discussed elsewhere in this book under 15 'Examples of influence that can steer even a meta-analysis of randomised controlled trials'. Making a drug look 'better' can mean it is made out to be more effective than the drug really is, which means a drug that is no better than a placebo is dressed up to look more effective(402) or made to appear safer than it really is.(403-405)

Apart from cheating, there is the simple but almost unsolvable problem of drug interactions. Many people take multiple drugs, and it is impossible to test for more than some interactions between them. As there is 'no evidence' for many interactions, even serious ones like a higher risk of heart attack or stroke can stay undiscovered for a long time. There is no solution to this conundrum apart from doctors' experience, intuition and a robust reporting system, but the point is that this is an example of a serious deficiency in the current system where intuitive judgment and heuristics could be very helpful and where a dose of humility is called for when advancing the idea that the current system is the only true way.

Even if a remedy is out of patent protection, it may only have a small market, so there are few companies or only one company producing that remedy. A favourite tactic has been to buy these companies and increase the price of the remedies, safe in the knowledge that even then even if there is no patent protection few or no competitors would bother to produce a competing remedy, as the approval process is too long and costly and the incumbent is free to reduce their price again if competition arises.

The tendency for unjustifiable price rises of pharmaceuticals has only recently been addressed, albeit partially, as some companies increased the price ten or fiftyfold.(406-408). It led to a political backlash and an announcement by the FDA that it will expedite applications for competing remedies in such cases, but it is unlikely that this will stop the less flagrant, ongoing abuse of this process where prices are raised.(409)

The How in Detail: Epidemiology and the Grading and Evaluation of Research Evidence

The hierarchy of evidence

Epidemiology has the following hierarchy of evidence such as the United States National Institute of Health (NIH)(410) or the Australian National Health and Medical Council (NHMRC)(411):

I	A systematic review of Level II studies
II	A randomised controlled trial
III-1	A pseudorandomised controlled trial (i.e. alternate allocation of some other method)
III-2	A comparative study with concurrent controls: • Non-randomised, experimental trial • Cohort study • Case-control study • Interrupted time series with a control group
III-3	A comparative study without concurrent controls: • Historical control study • Two or more single arm study • Interrupted time series without a parallel control group
IV	Case studies with either post-test or pre-test/post-test outcomes

Here as an image

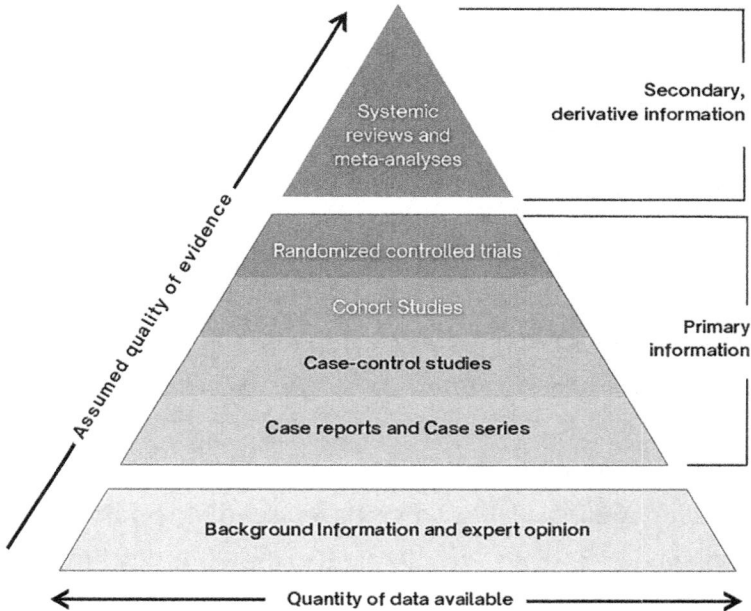

There are other, similar hierarchies such as the Cochrane hierarchy(410) that are also widely used.

In practice in most cases, in order to get regulators' approval to sell an intervention such as a pharmaceutical, randomised controlled trials are needed to show that the intervention has a worthwhile health effect.

The CONSORT 2010 statement and the ensuing corruption

The very widely adopted CONSORT 2010 statement provides guidelines and rules on how to report randomised controlled clinical trials.(187) It appears there is a general consensus that the Statement has improved the quality of the reporting of clinical trial results.

However, as explained below, in practice the CONSORT 2010 statement is also widely used as an instruction manual on how to misrepresent the true result of any clinical trial and how to set up clinical trials, so they provide the sought-after outcome for the sponsor of the trial.

That is similar to how the "Good Publication Practice" (GPP3) guidelines for industry-financed medical journal articles are being used as *a de facto manual for how marketing through academic journal content can be conducted in compliance with contemporary editorial standards"(412)*

The CONSORT 2010 statement has a very similar issue to evidence-based medicine. Evidence-based medicine has many individual success stories but during its reign population health is decreasing substantially. The CONSORT 2010 statement has led to better reporting of many clinical trials, but the authority provided by the Statement has been widely abused and misused making the reporting of many important clinical trials completely untrustworthy.

How is a statement that provides best practice reporting guidelines delivering the support for the exact opposite?

Below is an excerpt from the CONSORT 2010 statement itself defining the intent of the CONSORT 2010 statement, what the CONSORT 2010 statement does and does not do. The last sentence of the quote is part of the CONSORT 2010 statement:

> *"Diligent adherence by authors to the checklist items facilitates clarity, completeness, and transparency of reporting. Explicit descriptions, not ambiguity or*

omission, best serve the interests of all readers. Note that the CONSORT 2010 Statement does not include recommendations for designing, conducting, and analysing trials. It solely addresses the reporting of what was done and what was found."

A trial report that conforms to the CONSORT 2010 statement is given more credibility than a trial report that does not conform.

Anything ranging from billions of dollars to an individual promotion or an ability to continue working in the current role can depend on the outcome of a randomised controlled trial. As a consequence, the CONSORT 2010 statement has turned out to be a how-to guide to misrepresent, cheat, and lie about the efficacy of an intervention such as a cancer treatment when performing a randomised controlled trial while staying within the rules and being safe from the accusation of fraud.

As presented above the CONSORT 2010 statement itself declares:

> *"that the CONSORT 2010 Statement does not include recommendations for designing, conducting, and analysing trials. It solely addresses the reporting of what was done and what was found."*

This invites free rein to rampant lying. The lying simply has to happen in the design,(413) conduct, and analysis of the trial.

The lying also extends to the reporting of the trials as shown below.

Examples of such corruption together with reporting failures need not stop a trial being reported in a major journal such as New England Journal of Medicine (NEJM), Journal of the American Medical Association (JAMA), The Lancet, Nature and perhaps to a lesser degree in the British Medical Journal (BMJ) or Annals of Internal Medicine. Examples of both manipulation of the design, conduct and analysis of trials and also in the reporting, despite CONSORT 2010, include:

- choosing an outcome to measure that seems convincing but is misleading, such as level of cholesterol of oxygen levels instead of mortality;(414)
- changing the statistical methodology such as choosing a different endpoint (switching from, for example, mortality to the measurement of a biomarker);(139, 301, 302)
- testing an intervention that is materially different from the group that is expected to be treated, such as younger people with few or no comorbidities (other illnesses) compared to older people with multiple comorbidities that would be most of the future patients;(115, 415-420)
- underdosing, overdosing or mis-dosing the alternative remedy being compared;(260, 271, 301, 421, 422)
- running multiple trials and only reporting those that benefit the cause or reporting an unfavourable result late;(301, 413, 423, 424)
- excluding groups of trial participants;(139, 302)
- stopping a trial early or late when it suits;(414)
- running trials for marketing reasons or with substantial marketing input while stating that the trials were led by academics;(425)

- identify in a double or triple-blind study the patients receiving the active ingredient through the side-effects or other means and therefore being able to give those patients better care or excluding those among the group that received the active treatment with adverse outcomes;(302, 421)
- running many different analyses or even reporting results without giving evidence;(426)
- not reporting serious adverse events in publications, only to the regulator(427) and only reporting 3% to 33% of adverse events in the final publication while stating that all adverse events were recorded and only disclosing the true facts publicly two decades later;(428)
- not reporting conflicts of interests by the authors with conflicted authors typically providing more favourable results than unconflicted researchers;(429)
- giving the investigated treatment to the control group as well which leads to the discovery of long term effects being avoided to be recorded as that treatment eliminates the control group and makes comparisons impossible as happened in the trials of the mRNA COVID-19 vaccines;(430)
- deliberately or carelessly allowing the treatment to also be given to the control group during the trial, for example if the investigated treatment is commonly given by doctors in the area where the trial was conducted, if a non-result is desired;(421)
- authors receiving payments or being employed by organisations that have an interest in a particular outcome;(421, 424)
- and many, many other such methods that lead to the desired outcome.(431-433)

The manipulation can then be extended to meta-analyses of multiple trials that despite many flaws in their execution can still be published in a prestigious forum such as Nature(261) or Cochrane(261) if the result is suitable.

COVID-19 related clinical trials and their faults and qualities are covered at c19.org(238) and its many related webpages, all with "c19" in the URL.

In fact, pharmaceuticals can be described as 'a market for lemons' where the market produces lots of barely usable pills and devices that have lots of side effects and where deception is rife as a consequence of different levels of information being available for companies, regulators and consumers.(434, 435)

Hence the "*best*" run trials tend to be run by the people with the biggest stake in the outcome which are often pharmaceutical companies and therefore the best run trials are among the least credible. Financial disclosure, improving reporting standards and registering trials are not sufficient remedies.(436)

The power of the treatment guidelines, in deciding which interventions are to be used and paid for, created a very large incentive to game the creation of the guidelines by compromising the members of the panel and by gaming the research results used to create the guidelines by compromising the research evidence.(97-100, 109, 144-146, 437, 438)

Hence the rise of evidence-based medicine did not coincide with an increase in life expectancy beyond the rate of increase prevalent in 1995(20) and coincides with reduced life expectancy in the United States and other countries.

Tightening research standards

The usual response and perhaps the only response I have come across whenever evidence of malfeasance in medical research is discussed is to tighten research standards with some examples of a copious number of publications here.(439-444)

Tightening standards, including ethical standards, pre-trial reporting standards and post-trial reporting standards has effects that are worse than not tightening standards: Each additional standard increases the costs of research and therefore favours those with a large budget, i.e. those with the strongest motivation and the most power to compromise the system. Each additional standard also favours those who are least likely to come up with genuine new findings, which are the established incumbents.

Each additional rule and regulation make research harder for those who are genuinely looking for the new, the unexpected, the unknown but makes little difference to the motivated and those with deep pockets. Each additional rule and regulation create selective pressure to provide worse research.

Tightening ethical standards gives more power to ethical committees and therefore gives a veto to people who have the time to be on such committees, who may have professional jealousies and who can impose their own ideas on research, i.e. tightening standards makes research harder and more prone to interference and a force to stick to the known as researching the unknown will meet with more scepticism even though that is where the new findings are.(142)

Tightening pre-trial reporting standards and forcing trials to publish their chosen analysis and reporting methods has a number of pernicious effects, even when trials are also forced to always report their post-trial results. Such standards again make it harder to do entirely new research as the researchers simply do not know what will be worthwhile to report and therefore the researchers cannot say beforehand what of their research will be worth reporting, therefore favouring research into the known or premeditated and confirming what is already assumed to be correct rather than researching anything unknown. It also heavily favours incumbents as breakthrough research that replaces one or many interventions is less likely to happen, making the positions of incumbents less likely to be disrupted.

Those with sufficient funds have no major issue with pre- and post-trial reporting as they can simply invalidate a trial that is going wrong from their point of view by claiming that, for example, the randomisation of patients was done wrongly, or any of the active or control treatments was contaminated, or the double- or triple-blind veil was pierced or they stop a trial early or late or substitute an endpoint, i.e. trial result, with a more amenable one.

Consequences

Every stage in the creation of the "*best available evidence*" can and has been compromised and outright falsified despite the best efforts of many people to provide uncontaminated elements of the process of creating research results and medical treatment guidelines.

All of this has been amplified by the media, government agencies and governments themselves. Any one of these can create their own self-serving distortions if their ethical understanding allows them to do so and there is no absolute standard they are held to.

How could it come to such a catastrophical situation as we are having today?

It is clear that the financial beneficiaries from interventions have a strong incentive to adjust any system so that it favours them. A rule-based system such as epidemiology (the name of the science that underpins the research part of evidence-based medicine) is particularly easy to compromise as any lie is acceptable provided it conforms to the rules.

The outcome of the rules-based evidence-based medicine methodology has been so obviously bad on a population health and cost of healthcare level – with the United States the best example on getting the worst of both – that the question arises where is the demand coming from?

The demand comes from each of the components of billions of medical interactions each year:

- The financial beneficiaries of the interventions
- The patients, and
- The doctors.

There are no innocents in this.

Vested Interests Can Distort Science for a Long Time

It is well known that the tobacco lobby managed to forestall, reduce and influence government interventions against smoking for a long time by misusing the scientific process.(95, 222, 445)

Would the tobacco industry have been allowed to do this because so many people were still smoking in the 60s, 70s and 80s, i.e. was the pressure on tobacco companies smaller as there were many smokers who preferred to hear the lies of the tobacco companies than the fact that smoking was deeply harmful for their bodies? Without an audience, a liar is simply somebody holding forth in a pub.

The example of salt and cerebro-cardiovascular disease

Similar misuse is happening in the debate as to whether our current intake of sodium (table salt is sodium chloride) does or does not have an effect on cerebro-cardiovascular disease or all-cause mortality. In other words, do we eat so much salt that our chances of getting very sick or dying are increased?

I personally saw a presentation where the researcher showed that a Mediterranean diet led to better health outcomes than a Western diet. That finding was demolished by a senior member of the audience stating that the Mediterranean diet uses less salt, and this single fact could explain the difference in health outcomes. In other words, it seems received wisdom that more salt in a diet is harmful. That the Western diet is also heavier on sugar and starch and that may also be a confounder which means that sugar and starch may also affect the difference in health outcomes, was not mentioned.

Coming back to the benefits or otherwise of salt, to provide an overview of the state of knowledge in a particular field, there are either the Cochrane and other systematic reviews, which are discussed further down, or every once in a while, a scientist sits down to write a review of the current scientific evidence in a research field. Typically, this is a very knowledgeable person, and such reviews are sought after by those who are starting out in this field to give them an overview and a launching point. Hence, reviews are influential and can be a source of manipulation. This and other manipulations have been found in a review of reviews about sodium intake.(446)

It concludes that the debate about sodium is strongly polarised among those for and against reducing sodium with a third, smaller group in the middle.

This is a good case study to show how science can be and is being manipulated. If the truth is that sodium is either harmful or not harmful, then one of the two sides is likely manipulating the evidence. If the truth is that the evidence is inconclusive, then the two sides that come to a firm conclusion may both be manipulating the evidence.

There is a third possibility that sodium is harmful under some and beneficial or not harmful under other circumstances and that, despite much research, scientists are still unaware of these circumstances (confounders), but this scenario may become less and less likely the more trials are being conducted.

The first type of manipulation is that opposing evidence is ignored. From the above study:

> '• Published reports supporting either side of the
> hypothesis are less likely to cite contradictory
> papers.'

Systematic reviews either did a consistently bad job or were seemingly deliberately leaving out evidence that contradicted their conclusion:

> '• There was very little consistency in the selection
> of primary studies in systematic reviews on the
> topic.'

This could be interpreted as systematic reviewers either did not read previous reviews and did not do a good job searching for primary studies or that they deliberately left them out. As all systematic reviews suffered from this defect of selective reading, the first, more innocent explanation seems less likely to be true.

A few authors with strong views for either side dominated the publications, citations and the debate. Authors whose studies were inconclusive published fewer results and there were no dominant inconclusive authors.

There are major issues with the evidence. From the article:

> "(A) recent review of the methodological quality
> of observational studies relating sodium to
> cardiovascular outcomes found that methodological

defects, considered to have the potential to alter the direction of association, affected all 26 observational studies (except for one which showed a null association)"(447) as quoted in.(446)

The review of reviews above did not mention the word 'industry' once. It is much cheaper to produce well-tasting food by using plenty of salt and there is evidence that salt has addictive qualities when used in the 'right' proportions.(126) Hence there is a strong financial incentive for processed food manufacturers to downplay any evidence of sodium causing harm. Equally, this could then lead to the opposing side, in reaction, gilding the lily the other way.

Subversion of the scientific process

There is plenty of evidence that the scientific process can be subverted for at least a few decades by vested interests, even for subjects that are vital to public health. Likely examples are osteoporosis, cholesterol, painkillers, antidepressants, medical guidelines, diet, diabetes, obesity (chapter 12 and elsewhere in(91)) and sugar.(123) This is a sharp indictment for the reliability of evidence-based medicine, seeing the 'evidence' can be manipulated for such a long time. The truth can be extensive and detailed, for example, sodium may be right on the edge of being harmful or not harmful, but it is the job of science to discern the truth and therefore to find out if and when sodium is or is not harmful and to clearly state so if science is unable to discern the truth.

Decreasing population health by reducing fat and increasing sugar consumption

The research that has probably been most damaging to population health in the last 50 years consists of two randomised controlled studies that laid the foundation for the belief that saturated fats were worse than unsaturated fats and lower fat diets were healthier than high fat diets.

The first is the 1966 to 1973 Sydney Diet Heart Study and the second is the Minnesota Coronary Experiment from 1968 to 1973. In both cases, substituting unsaturated fat (Omega 6 linoleic acid) for animal fats rich in saturated fatty acids led to a reduction in blood cholesterol but an increase in all-cause deaths and deaths from cardiovascular disease and coronary heart disease in the Sydney Diet Heart Study(80) and to a 22% higher risk of death for each 30mg/dl (0.78 mmol/L) in serum cholesterol reduction in the Minnesota Coronary Experiment.(81)

The original authors of the studies did not mention the changes in mortality, only the reduction in serum cholesterol which led to firstly saturated fats and then all fats being discouraged *despite the fact that such a diet increased mortality.*

A team of researchers re-investigated the original raw data, publishing their results in 2013 and 2016,(80, 81) so the above has only recently become known – more than 40 years after the end of the original studies.

How can this happen? One reason could have been that it was much harder to do the statistical calculations in the early 1970s, as statistics itself was less developed and computers were much slower and, for example, used punch cards but mortality is just as easy to record as cholesterol levels.

To reduce costs, many randomised controlled trials do not measure mortality or morbidity directly, which are usually rarer events requiring large trials, but concentrate on a so-called intermediate marker that is considered a good indicator for future mortality or morbidity. At the time it made perfect sense to use blood cholesterol level as just such an intermediate marker that could be used as a substitute for future mortality and morbidity and the original researchers may then not have looked very hard for changes in mortality and morbidity.

As was the prevailing opinion then and, to this author's knowledge even now, the most plausible outcome of a reduction in blood cholesterol levels would have been a reduction in mortality and morbidity(437, 448-452) but, surprisingly, this did not happen in these long-running trials and the researchers chose not to publish the mortality and morbidity data.(78, 453)

In addition, if those trials would have been run today, their result could have been just as misleading. The most powerful way to control statistical abuse at the moment is to register a randomised controlled trial in advance, typically with a government-run clinical trial register and in the case of those two trials, they would have registered that they are looking for reduced blood cholesterol levels and would have succeeded.

In other words, 50 years of tightening research standards still would not have uncovered the abuse of not reporting an unexpected counter intuitive result such as reduced cholesterol but increased death and illness rates.

The evidence of those two trials is therefore more indicative of cholesterol having a protective effect as increased cholesterol is associated with lower mortality.(448, 451, 454)

How could such an abuse happen as it did in those two trials? Only a very small number of people – the statisticians in the original study – would have been in a position to realise what happened. Other members of the trial team with intimate knowledge of the data may have suspected something but, as the rates of death and illness were not much larger, the statisticians could have easily overridden any objections, especially as reporting the full truth would have replaced a very important result (reduced blood cholesterol levels) with a non-result – a change in the type of fat consumption makes no difference to your death or illness rates or, worse even, a change in the type of fat consumption increases morbidity and mortality.

These two trials are an excellent example to show in detail what is wrong with evidence-based medicine. They ticked and still do tick all the right boxes, and the impact has been devastating to population health; furthermore, the devastation is continuing:

The two studies led to the food industry being allowed, in fact supported by government, to advertise fat reduced but sugar increased processed foods as being healthy – a great financial boon as animal fats (saturated fats) are more expensive than unsaturated fats which are more expensive than sugar. Hence, the food industry could sell cheaper processed food as being healthier than more expensive existing food.

When misleading research leads to government recommendations which coincide with commercial interests, it can lead to quite serious damage to the health of the population as it did and still does in this case. There are for example still very few if any extra taxes on sugary drinks that are consumed in vast numbers and cause serious damage to population health.(82-84, 123, 124)

Any evaluation of the benefits and effectiveness of evidence-based medicine needs to take major population health disasters like these into account.

> These trials were large scale randomised controlled trials run by reputable people over years, yet their results were and are highly damaging.

The common rejoinder that the system works as the truth has eventually been uncovered ignores that this truth is not public policy and may not be for a long time yet. Meanwhile, damage continues to be caused by wrong government policy recommendations and bad quality but highly profitable processed food being sold. There is some movement in the stance from government agencies but the process is very slow, as this article from The Economist shows.(455)

It is also not part of a medical doctor's training how much food and drink affect health nor how to use diet to improve patients' and population health. Only in 2024 was an extensively researched bestseller published by a medical doctor, Casey Means that covers how to improve health through what a person takes into their body.(456) There have been many best selling books on diet and health before but for the first time with the elevation of Robert F. Kennedy to lead the United States Department of Health, a cabinet position is there a person ready to take action to reverse the current decline in population health.

CHAPTER 11

SCIENTIFIC PUBLISHING:
FINANCIAL ISSUES, INDEXING OF PUBLICATIONS, REJECTION RATES, PEER REVIEW AND PROPOSED REMEDIES

Introduction

Evidence-based medicine needs medical research results to be published in book form or as articles in scientific journals in order to adopt the findings from those research results. Scientific publishing is an odd beast.

It is hugely profitable for the publishers. In the past it was very difficult to get to read scientific papers unless you had an employer or were associated with a university with a library that subscribed to the relevant journals and even then, full access might have been limited to a few people. Today this has eased a little, but it is still impossible to do a comprehensive review without institutional access or without the funds to pay $30-40 each for a raft of papers or to access a site that gives illegal access to scientific publications.

Scientific publishers have net profit margins around and above 30% of turnover, an otherwise rare percentage for large companies. Reed Elsevier for example, the biggest publisher, gained STG2.2 billion on revenues of STG7.2 billion in 2021, a profit margin of 31%.

These issues of costs to do medical research are well known and there are strong movements aimed at making scientific publications more accessible.

The importance of prestige

The underlying problem is that scientific articles are in large part evaluated by where they are published, i.e. in how prestigious a publication they appear. A prestigious journal like Nature, Cell, the British Medical Journal, the Lancet or the New England Journal of Medicine gives a substantial boost to a researcher's career. As such, papers also boost the universities' reputation and a bounty paid by government to a researcher for a paper in Nature can be as high as $165,000(457) in the case of the Chinese government.

There has been one significant change in recent years as much searching for articles is either done in specialised databases like PubMed or Web of Science; PubMed has the benefit that searches are repeatable – the same search done by different people on different computers comes up with identical results, unlike the main free alternative, Google Scholar. Google Scholar potentially shows different results for the same search every time that search is made but it weighs them in part by the number of citations. Some researchers concluded that it may be the more useful tool and may have been so since 2013(458) but this currently seems a minority view.

Reasons for considering Google Scholar of less value as a research tool include that a lot of publications are of questionable scientific merit and a lot of the citations are of lower value than the citations counted in commercial databases like Embase or Scopus, as Google's definition of a citation is much wider. Google Scholar seems to make little use of the prestige of a publication and the number of citations seems to be more important in its sorting algorithm and in what then goes to the top of a Google Scholar search.

The rise of Google Scholar, with its lower emphasis on the prestige of the journal, does not seem to have made a difference to the demand by scientists to be published in the more prestigious journal. As an example, rejection rates in journals associated with the American Psychological Association are on average 76% and range up to 91%. Prestigious journals have rejection rates in the 90% range which means that they reject at least nine out of ten publications submitted.

Peer review

Almost all reputable scientific journals use a process called peer review to evaluate a newly submitted paper as explained well here.(459) An often unpaid editor receives a manuscript and decides whether it is worth taking further. If the answer is yes that paper is then submitted to one or more always unpaid peer reviewers who are asked for their usually anonymous opinion about it.

The many weaknesses of this process, like competitors of the researcher evaluating a paper, reviewers plagiarising and simultaneously rejecting a paper, reviewers doing a poor or very poor job due to lack of time and or relevant expertise, reviews being little different from chance and so on are well known, as outlined by Richard Smith(460), a former editor of the British Medical Journal (BMJ), one of the most respected scientific journals. His conclusion is:

> *"So peer review is a flawed process, full of easily identified defects with little evidence that it works. Nevertheless, it is likely to remain central to science and journals because there is no obvious alternative, and scientists and editors have a continuing belief in peer review.* **How odd that science should be rooted in belief***."*

The same author in 2010(461) quotes one of his colleagues, Douglas Rennie, thus:

> *"there seems to be no study too fragmented, no hypothesis too trivial, no literature too biased or too egotistical, no design too warped, no methodology too bungled, no presentation of results too inaccurate, too obscure, and too contradictory, no analysis too self-serving, no*

*argument too circular, no conclusions too trifling
or too unjustified, and no grammar and syntax too
offensive for a paper to end up in print."*

That is actually excellent news as it means that even weird and wonderful papers can get into print and the censorship exercised by tightening research standards is not complete. It also means that if a research finding is not mainstream, whether true or not, it has a chance to be published.

The same publication lists a number of studies outlining the weaknesses of peer reviews: It can take months or years for a study to be published – this is on top of the time it takes to do ethics applications, do the study and write it up. These delays are costly, as they push up the costs of research and, concluding from the above, the peer review process may not add value as it can largely be a lottery, as the likelihood of agreement among peer reviewers is only slightly more than chance.

It is worth considering what it actually means that no single individual (peer reviewer) seems to be able to evaluate the scientific quality of a study from those studies that pass an editor's quality control. Does that mean that only the editor adds value to the process? The author has not found research that evaluates what value an editor adds to the process of scientific publishing.

The same article by Richard Smith also shows that peer reviewers have very little ability to spot even obvious, albeit unexpected errors and that they are biased – a group of scientists re-submitted 12 published papers authored by members of prestigious institutions to the same high-status journals in which the original papers had been published with changes in the titles, abstracts and introductions of the original publications but purportedly coming from no-name institutions. Three journals spotted the duplicates, eight of the remaining nine were rejected. Clearly, the researchers could have selected 12 particularly bad studies that, surprisingly, had passed muster in the past. If that was not the case, then a likely answer is that peer reviewers have a bias towards prestigious institutions, which would be completely understandable as peer review is unpaid and it would make sense that papers from prestigious institutions are more likely to be worth publishing. However, is using heuristics (mental shortcuts) like these science?

As peer review has aspects of a lottery, there are many highly original papers from future Nobel prize winners and other breakthroughs that failed peer review repeatedly.(462)

Interestingly, as the article by Richard Smith further describes, training peer reviewers, not disclosing the name of authors to peer reviewers and making peer reviewers' names public have not made much difference. I have had a paper reviewed by a public peer reviewer and the review felt worse than the substantial number of anonymous reviews I received as I experienced that person playing to the gallery rather than looking at the actual paper's content.

The demand for more and more scientific journals

For an author, one common way to deal with this process of publications is to submit their article to progressively less prestigious publications until peer review favours them.

One outcome of this process is that there is a demand for scientific journals that are less and less selective in the articles they publish. Hence the rise of so-called predatory journals that engage in little or no peer review.

Another development in scientific publishing is 'open access publishing'. In normal scientific publishing the author pays nothing for publication, but the reader has to subscribe to the journal or pay, typically $30-40 per article to read that article if they only want a specific article. In open access publishing, where an open access journal can be very prestigious and owned by a major scientific publisher, the author pays, typically about $1,500-5,000 or in some cases even more, per article, and the reader gets access to the article for free. An interesting discussion of the cost of both forms of publishing can be found here.(463) Overall, by 2024, open access has become much more prevalent, which makes research substantially easier though the evidence whether open access leads to more citations is inconclusive.(464) All publishers, whether closed or open source give access to Google Scholar to index their papers.

When you consider the difficulties with peer review and the phenomenon of open access publishing, a number of people spotted a business opportunity of creating journals with impressive titles or titles very similar to high-status journals, that accept just about every paper, thereby undermining trust in the process of scientific publishing altogether.

A librarian and associate professor at the University of Colorado, Jeffrey Beall, published an annual Beall's list of what he considers to be fake scientific publications. His 2016 list had 882 journals on it with this number having grown from 507 in 2015 and 303 in 2014.(465) He has since stopped publishing and de-clared that his university is investigating him for misconduct, moved to another library and retired in 2018. His work has been taken up by commercial enterprises which do not make their results publicly available. Many universities do not pay for the services of these commercial enterprises but exhort their re-searchers to be discerning, though there are many examples of researchers publishing in journals that are fake or border-line fake.(466)

In other words, it seems that the process of scientific publish-ing has major issues both for top and less prestigious journals. A systematic review of the effects of editorial peer review con-cluded that, 'Editorial peer review, although widely used, is largely untested and its effects are uncertain'.(467)

In one way, the selection effect of journals is very clear. Research that supports the approved narrative of COVID-19 was easy to publish in the most prestigious journals while research that went counter was limited to much less prestigious journals. This can be observed in detail on c19ivm.org and its sister web pages where many of the studies published in major scientific journals are excoriated for their lack of truthfulness.(40, 468)

Science Rooted in Belief

If "*science is rooted in belief*"(460), then evidence-based medicine is based on belief. We can argue that the latter does not need to be perfect and that it is enough to know that evidence-based medicine is the best form of medicine available – but what are the conclusions to be drawn here, especially as the output of evidence-based medicine is as flawed and as open to manipulation as it is?

With such a weak foundation, are we truly in a position to claim that evidence-based medicine is superior to all other forms of medicine and are we truly in a position to claim that it should be the dominant or only form of medicine that should be practised?

There is clearly substantiation that evidence-based medicine works better in certain areas than tradition, experience, intuition and expert consensus. However, is there evidence that it works better often enough or even evidence that its advantages outweigh the disadvantages?

The research method employed by evidence-based medicine should come with a serious health warning: *"May or may not be true, may or may not be useful, may or may not create more problems than it solves, use with caution."*

Proposed Remedies

Proposed remedies for the poor quality of published research try to improve the quality of individual research results by increasing transparency: *"Make publicly available the full protocols, analysis plans or sequence of analytical choices, and raw data for all designed and undertaken biomedical research,"* by pre-registering trials, increasing training of researchers and rewarding researchers who make reproduction easier.(442)

These measures sound like common sense and many of them have been enshrined in a set of recommended research practices called CONSORT, with the latest being CONSORT 2010.(187) as written about in the previous chapter.

One impression when reading CONSORT 2010 is that it seems to have been written without regard to the costs of the many proposals and it does not set any priorities – the assumption is that researchers should adhere to all the reporting requirements in full. It is as if in car design it was just as important to have a fully working ashtray as to have fully working headlights, brakes and air bags.

Another proposal is to not just present 'good results' but also to present results that were inconclusive or where no effect was measured, so researchers have a more complete picture. A quote from the field of preclinical cancer studies: "*There must be more opportunities to present negative data.*"(444) This makes sense but a so-called literature review of the existing publications in a field can already take many months. An evaluation of the benefit versus the costs of having to review many more publications may be worthwhile. This information load may become more manageable by employing artificial intelligence tools.

I am not providing links to such tools as artificial intelligence is in the middle of an expectation and spending boom with very rapid shifts and any tool that may be the best today could be superseded within weeks

A further proposal is not to give primacy to objective improvements but to consider subjective improvements as well, which means that treatments are considered worthwhile even if they do not improve the health of the patient but make the patient feel better. This approach is much favoured by alternative practitioners and even by established researchers with roots in the alternative practitioner movement.(469) However, this is a minority view and achieving both objective and subjective improvements together seems to be a more worthwhile pursuit. That dual approach is implied by the term 'clinical significance', i.e. a finding that is significant enough to be used in clinical (medical) practice.

If a scientific finding is meant to be true, it is meant to be reproducible. However, to quote Begley et al(441):

> "In biomedical research, we are in the midst of a revolution with the generation of new data and scientific publications at a previously unprecedented rate. However, unfortunately, there is compelling evidence that the majority of these discoveries will not stand the test of time."

and

> "Over the recent years, there has been an increasing recognition of the weaknesses that pervade our current system of basic and preclinical research. This has been highlighted empirically in preclinical research by the inability to replicate the majority of findings presented in high-profile journals. The estimates for irreproducibility based on these empirical observations range from 75% to 90%. These estimates fit remarkably well with estimates of 85%(440, 443, 470-473) for the proportion of biomedical research that is wasted at-large. This irreproducibility is not unique to preclinical

studies. It is seen across the spectrum of biomedical research. For example, similar concerns have been expressed for observational research where zero of 52 predictions from observational studies were confirmed in randomized clinical trials."

Incidentally, if zero of 52 predictions turned out to be true, then it is statistically unlikely that more than 7% of all observations are true. Technically, the upper end of the 95% confidence interval is around 0.07 with minor variations depending on the assumed distribution. In Stata, a statistical software, the command is 'cii prop 52 0'.

What does the above paragraph mean? Statistics has a way to deal with the following effect: If you toss a coin once and it shows up as 'heads' then you have not enough coin tosses to decide whether the coin is biased (more likely to show heads or tails) or not. If you toss the coin three times and they are all heads, that is still a common event for an unbiased coin. If you toss the coin ten times and they are all heads, it is now more likely than not that the coin is biased. If the first twenty tosses are all heads you can become quite certain as the chance of that happening with an unbiased coin (twenty heads or twenty tails in a row) are only two in a million.

The next question is then how biased the coin is and here statistics is helpful using what is called the binomial distribution. Similar to the above, if you make 52 predictions (as a type of coin toss, a prediction may inherently have a much higher or lower chance of success if chosen at random) and none of the 52 predictions are correct, then your true ability to make correct predictions is most likely somewhere between 0% and

7% and less likely to be more than 7%. In other words, since none of the predictions from the 52 observational trials were true, it is less likely that more than 7% (or 4 or more out of 52) of predictions from observational studies turn out to be true and it is quite possible that predictions from observational studies of the type evaluated are never or hardly ever true, or, as ever, the source from where this information comes needs to be evaluated for reliability as other research concluded that observational studies are not inferior to randomised controlled trials, with a lively, ongoing discussion among researchers underway.(474-480)

CHAPTER 12

THE FOUNDATIONS OF EVIDENCE-BASED MEDICINE

Why Is Evidence-based Medicine Important?

E vidence-based medicine is defined and explained in detail below and is the standard way that medicine is practised today. *"In the UK, for example, it is now a contractual requirement for all doctors, nurses and pharmacists to practise (and for managers to manage) according to best research evidence."*(119)

A 1997 study, which does not seem to have been repeated, showed a large rise in the number of medical articles that refer to evidence-based medicine.(140) Evidence-based medicine has certainly had an influence on public policy(481) and anecdotally it is considered to be dominant in clinical practice via guidelines.

Evidence-based medicine is important as it is the dominant and enforced paradigm on how to practise medicine.

What Is Evidence-based Medicine?

In the full Oxford English Dictionary(482) *"evidence"* is defined as *'Ground for belief; testimony or facts tending to prove or disprove any conclusion'* with a quote from the 1809 Medical & Physical Journal: *"The truth of which I can yet attest by living evidence".*

The *"simple definition of evidence"* in the Merriam-Webster dictionary is *"something which shows that something else exists or is true"*, and other dictionaries link evidence and truth.

Evidence-based medicine is defined by David Sackett(118), the person most identified with the founding and popularising of evidence-based medicine, in the Encyclopedia of Biostatistics. (483) Reading that definition, evidence-based medicine is a dream come true for the clinician – the definition is reproduced here in detail because of how much these paragraphs differ from today's practice of evidence-based medicine:

> *"In this definition, the practice of evidence-based medicine means integrating individual clinical expertise with a critical appraisal of the best available external clinical evidence from systematic research. By individual clinical expertise is meant the proficiency and judgment that individual clinicians acquire through clinical experience and clinical practice.*

Increased expertise is reflected in many ways, but especially in more effective and efficient diagnosis and in the more thoughtful identification and compassionate use of individual patients' predicaments, rights, and preferences in making clinical decisions about their care.

By best available external clinical evidence is meant clinically relevant research, often from the basic sciences of medicine, but especially from patient-centered clinical research into the accuracy and precision of diagnostic tests (including the clinical examination), the power of prognostic factors, and the efficacy and safety of therapeutic, rehabilitative, and preventive regimens."(484)

The entire entry is worth reading because it is very convincing. Evidence-based medicine is described as:

"The practice of evidence-based medicine is a process of lifelong, self-directed learning in which caring for one's own patients creates the need for clinically important information about diagnosis, prognosis, therapy, and other clinical and health care issues, and in which its practitioners:

1. Convert these information needs into answerable questions.

2. Track down, with maximum efficiency, the best evidence with which to answer them (and making increasing use of secondary sources of the best evidence). Examples of such secondary sources are the Cochrane Library and journals of critically appraised clinical articles such as ACP Journal Club and Evidence-based medicine.

3. Critically appraise that evidence for its validity **(closeness to the truth)** *and usefulness (clinical applicability).*

4. Integrate the appraisal with clinical expertise and apply the results in clinical practice.

5. Evaluate one's own performance."(ibid.)

Clearly, this might be what good doctors are already doing, and the process is simplified by the research evaluation replaced by guidelines. The nod to evidence being evaluated for "*closeness to the truth*" is also reassuring.

Evidence-based treatments are happening elsewhere as well according to David Sackett:

"Parallel developments, still with the individual patient as the focus of attention, are occurring in other clinical disciplines (evidence-based surgery, evidence-based nursing, evidence-based dentistry, etc.). Other evidence-based disciplines consider the community as the focus of attention rather than the individual patient (evidence-based public health), or add an explicit economic element and seek to purchase or provide that mix of health care that will

maximize some group or public benefit (evidence-based purchasing)."(118)

Evidence-based medicine can be done according to David Sackett in the same publication:

"Recent audits in the front lines of clinical care have documented that some inpatient clinical teams in general medicine,(485) psychiatry(486) and surgery (P. McCulloch, personal communication) have provided evidence-based care to the vast majority of their patients. Such studies show that busy clinicians who devote their scarce reading time to selective, efficient, patient-driven searching, appraisal and incorporation of the best available evidence can practise evidence-based medicine."

Once evidence-based medicine was defined, it needed a scientific basis. That scientific basis seems a bit shaky:

The two references in the previous quote are both authored by David Sackett.

In the first reference(485) cited by David Sackett a team of clinicians in a hospital analysed what they did for 109 treatments and classified 53% as supported by randomised controlled trial and for a further 29% there was unanimity about the existence of convincing non-experimental evidence; in other words, the treatment was obvious like antibiotics for sepsis or extensive cellulitis. 18% of their work was non-evidence-based like antacids and reassurance for non-cardiac chest pain and specific symptomatic and supportive care for people close to death or mild or late poisonings. This article was in response to quoted accusations that only 10-20% of the treatments they provide have any scientific foundation which originated from a statement on page 5 of this 1985 (United States) National Academy of Sciences report.(487)

The first reference cited by Sackett(485) does not directly contradict the stated percentage for individual treatments but contradicts this number when you look at each patient. In other words, patients may receive a mix of treatments, but the large majority receive some form of evidence-based treatment.

However, in a British Medical Journal editorial by Tricia Greenhalgh, a famous populariser of evidence-based medicine, the limitations of such studies was exposed(488):

> *"A survey which addressed the question 'Is my practice evidence-based?' and which fulfilled all these criteria would be a major and highly expensive undertaking"*

i.e., Sackett's study was insufficient evidence. Further details as to why *"the impressive percentages obtained in these series should be interpreted cautiously"* are provided in that British Medical Journal article.(488)

The second reference cited by Sackett (evidence-based care in psychiatry(486)) consists of a conference presentation that is not easily available for download.

Evidence-based Medicine in Practice

Below David Sackett(118) deals with objections.

Firstly, he deals with the objection that judgment will be replaced by rules – he denies that judgment will be replaced by rules:

> *"Common misconceptions about evidence-based medicine include the concern that it might degenerate into 'cookbook' medicine. However, because it requires a bottom-up approach that integrates the best external evidence with individual clinical expertise and patient choice, it cannot result in slavish, cookbook approaches to individual patient care.*
>
> *External clinical evidence can inform, but can never replace, individual clinical expertise, and it is this expertise that decides whether the external evidence applies to the individual patient at all and, if so, how it should be integrated into a clinical decision.*
>
> *Similarly, any external guideline must be integrated with individual clinical expertise in deciding whether and how it matches the patient's clinical state, predicament, and preferences, and thus whether it should be applied. Clinicians who fear top-down cookbooks will find the advocates of evidence-based medicine joining them at the barricades."*

In practice, external clinical evidence does a lot more than *"inform ... individual clinical expertise"*. The best protection from malpractice suits, loss of employment and regulatory scrutiny is following the evidence-based guidelines issued to doctors even though much of these guidelines are produced by doctors who receive payments from the pharmaceutical industry.(91)

Secondly Professor Sackett, as stated the founder or one of the main popularisers of evidence-based medicine deals with the objection that evidence-based medicine will be used to cut costs:

> *"Others fear that evidence-based medicine will be hijacked by purchasers and managers to cut the costs of health care. This would not only be a misuse of evidence-based medicine but suggests a fundamental misunderstanding of its financial consequences. Doctors practicing evidence-based medicine will identify and apply the most efficacious interventions to maximize the quality and quantity of life for individual patients; this may raise rather than lower the cost of their care."*

Sackett was correct about the increased costs – healthcare 20 years later costs society some 80% more. However, also 20 years later, an excess of rules is precisely what had happened by then and evidence-based medicine has been hijacked by pharmaceutical companies.(60, 91, 120, 221, 489) Once evidence has become particularly valuable, including financially valuable, is it surprising that those who benefit from this process, for example vendors of treatments, have a strong incentive to provide evidence that supports their favoured treatment with possibly less regard for the underlying truth?

Key points to consider are that:

1. **evidence-based medicine substitutes <u>rules</u> for truth, experience and intuition and;**
2. **evidence-based medicine substitutes the quest for truth, intuition and the healing of the patient with <u>a quest to fulfil rules</u>.**

That is how evidence-based medicine is practised with the guideline writers tasked with how close the evidence is to the truth. In practice, that evaluation of closeness to the truth is how much the evidence conforms to the rules even assuming there is no corruption involved in the writing of the guidelines.

A clinician who accepts evidence-based medicine as the dominant theme of their practice has made the error of accepting that rules are dominating their practice, thinking along the lines of:

"If there are randomised trials (possibly weighed by meta-analyses), then I will accept that this treatment is worth incorporating into my practice."

The crucial part is that this statement is very different from:

"If there are randomised trials (possibly weighed by meta-analyses), then I will consider accepting that this treatment is worth incorporating into my practice provided my judgment and intuition agree."

The first statement allows clinical practice to be manipulated by vested interests, the second statement is harder to control.

Leaving treatments to the judgments of physicians will mean that there are lots of faulty judgments made – humans make errors all the time – but such a system is more robust against being hijacked by vested interests. Errors are made by individuals on individuals, not system wide.

As gatekeepers for very large amounts of spending, doctors and other health professionals are a highly attractive target for manipulation as shown in the second half of chapter six of Akerlof and Shiller's book.(490) The moment doctors let rules dominate their judgment they can be manipulated on an industrial scale.

David Sackett's point that clinicians should use evidence to supplement their judgment is obvious and valuable, but evidence is now dominating judgment to the detriment of clinicians and patients. **The clinicians have lost a substantial amount of control, and the patients are being treated less as individuals and more as statistics.**

<u>As stated, evidence-based medicine's deepest flaw in practice is that it is not about truth or people, but about rules.</u>

Does Evidence-based Medicine Work?

The benefits of evidence-based medicine are many as one could count the results of all scientific medical research as being part of evidence-based medicine. It gets less clear when we compare evidence-based medicine with what came before it, which was expert scientific opinion despite such a process disparagingly being described as *"good old boys sat around a table"*.(119)

It may take a long time for a doctor to see enough patients with a particular range of symptoms for that practitioner to come to a reliable judgment based on experience. In such cases, evidence-based medicine has been particularly helpful. Examples are: designing many clinical guidelines about asthma and other ailments, discovering clinical trial data that is unreliable, improving awareness of the dangers of over-diagnosing certain ailments, exposing hospitals for bad practice, finding useful infectious diseases and many other treatments, post-surgery complications(120) and the Cochrane collaboration that created reliable systematic reviews of clinical trials(121) before it got usurped by vested interests.(491-493)

The Effect of Evidence-based Medicine

Evidence-based medicine has worked well in improving the effectiveness of many medical interventions or treatments. Evidence-based medicine has been able to improve the life expectancy of those diagnosed with cancer but unable to reduce the *increase* in the (age adjusted) rate of cancer, which is the statistical expectation of an individual to have cancer during their life.(214) With worldwide ageing populations this means that despite evidence-based medicine there has been a very strong rise in the number of cancer diagnoses.

This paper(494) shows that the cumulative lifetime risk of cancer in the first 85 years of life in Britain has gone up by 7% (men) and 11% (women) for those born in 1960 compared to those born in 1930. As smoking rates in the United States for example dropped from 42.4% of adults in 1965 to 16.8% in 2014,(495) that increase – instead of an expected decrease in cancer rates – is surprising.

If you feel that it is unfair to blame evidence-based medicine for not reducing the rate of cancer in the population, or just to stop the unexpected increase in the rate of cancer described above, consider the vast amounts of money that have been spent on evidence-based research for cancer alone which, on the other hand, has confirmed and furthered our knowledge that it is possible to reduce the rate of cancer, provided people change their lifestyles. However, evidence-based medicine has been unable to provide the information on *how* to implement this knowledge in practice and the amount spent on how to prevent the occurrence of cancer(496, 497) is much smaller than the spending on diagnostics and treatments and there are also imbalances with research spending not in proportion to the burden on society.(498)

The misallocation of resources and attention caused by the rise of evidence-based medicine as clinical trial results are limited in their applicability to individual patients and the near complete emphasis on pharmaceuticals and medical devices leaving much else of medicine in an evidence vacuum and the need for industry sponsorship have been pointed out by others.(121)

In other words, vast sums of money have been spent on acquiring knowledge that has not been useful in that evidence-based medicine has not provided a mechanism to translate that knowledge into behavioural changes in the population that leads to greater population health. This means that the strongest influence on health in industrialised nations, patient behaviour, has not been substantially addressed or improved by evidence-based medicine.

The question is, why not? Why has this immense amount of money not translated into reduced cancer rates? What is missing in evidence-based medicine that this seemingly simple step has so far been impossible for it to take?

As we can see, there are major benefits but there are also major issues with evidence-based medicine itself as it replaces experience and the art of healing and intuition with a set of rules. Rules can and do get manipulated by vested interests like those that are providing interventions, with the pharmaceutical industry an obvious example.

Rules also allow a bureaucracy to control doctors through regulations.

The absence of a rule that population health outcomes should have a high priority when funding and evaluating medical research means that population health outcomes are not given sufficient priority leading to the catastrophic outcomes we are observing today.

Another question that arises is:

Are we, as a society, overall better off with the rise of evidence-based medicine and therefore, do the benefits outweigh the disadvantages? I could not find any research answering this question.

A further question that arises is:

What is the relationship between the 'evidence' in evidence-based medicine and truth?

Putting it very mildly, this relationship may in practice not be as straightforward as it looks, especially when we start thinking that the only way to discern truth is through evidence.

CHAPTER 13

INHERENT CORRUPTION
IN THE RESEARCH PROCESS AND STATISTICS IS NOT A SETTLED SCIENCE

Introduction

Research happens under conditions and circumstances that encourage corruption, i.e. it is easier to provide false evidence than evidence that is true as there are many ways to create evidence that lead to false results but that are acceptable by the system even after scrutiny. Examples are mis-dosing or mis-timing the control treatment, using a placebo as control rather than best practice, plus the many other measures highlighted in this book.

An even deeper issue is that the actual tools used in statistics are very limited and can lead to wildly different results even when different statisticians sincerely look at the same dataset.

This chapter will first offer an example of statistics giving very different results when wielded by different researchers and then a number of examples of why it is easier or more beneficial for the researchers to provide results that are either knowingly false or are unlikely to be true or where it is very uncertain whether the results are true.

Statistics Is Not a Settled Science

Even a very simple-looking scientific question will be answered in many different ways by different scientists. In a famous example, three researchers gathered 61 scientists who collaborated in 29 groups with each group working on the same problem(499): *Are referees in soccer (football) more likely to give red cards to dark- skinned players?*

The 29 groups came up with 29 different answers with 69% saying that there is a statistically significant difference and 31% saying that there is not, as this chart shows. Another example of this chart are shown on fivethirtyeight.com, an at the time election- and, more relevantly, sport-oriented website here: (500, 501)

The authors of this study quite carefully worked on finding and, where possible, eliminating any errors that led to different results. Each group of scientists submitted their draft solution and each group's summary and analytic approach were given to all the other groups.

Identical Data, Different Conclusions

Twenty-nine teams of qualified researchers received the same set of football (soccer) data and were requested to find out if referees are more likely to give red cards to dark-skinned players. No prompts were given on what statistical methods to use. No team used the same method. Each team had a different result even though each team knew about all other approaches.

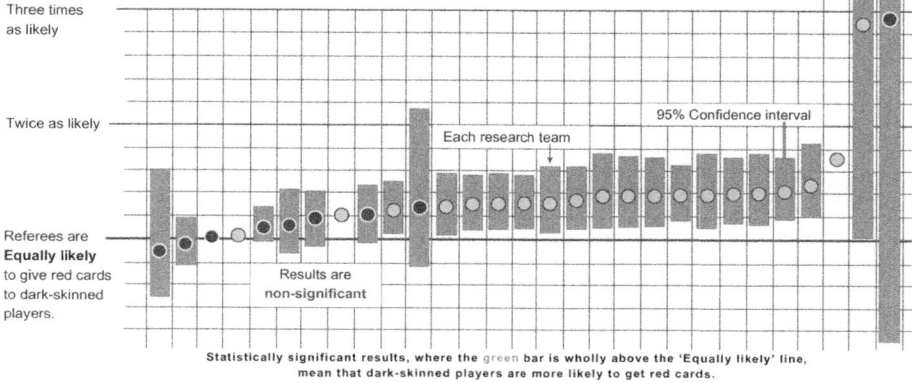

Statistically significant results, where the green bar is wholly above the 'Equally likely' line, mean that dark-skinned players are more likely to get red cards.

Each group was then asked to give feedback on at least three approaches and an opinion of how confident they were in that particular approach. This feedback was combined and then given out to all.

Everybody then submitted their final analysis, and a further round of feedback was given, this time with each team knowing not just the other teams' approaches but also their results. This led to further changes.

The main reasons why each team provided a different result is because they chose different statistical models (different statistical tools to analyse the data) and because they included or excluded certain variables like 'player position', such as striker or defender.

In an email discussion I had with other statisticians about this study, the argument was made that in a well-designed randomised controlled trial there would be much less variation in the outcome as it would be clearer which variable to include or exclude. However, 'well-designed' may not be a settled term among statisticians as in this study 29 teams used 29 analytic approaches – from the very simple to the very complex. It is possible to do something very similar, using lots of different approaches, with randomised controlled trials, including the amount of manipulation of randomised controlled trials that is actually happening and *"even a totally unbiased, perfectly randomized, reliably blinded, and faithfully executed clinical trial may still generate false and irreproducible results"*(167)

The 61 scientists were mostly highly qualified with 38 having a PhD and 17 a Master's degree *"and 24 have published at least one methodological/statistical article"*.

Did the more highly qualified teams better understand how to analyse the data than the less highly qualified ones? The answer was no – the results of both groups were equally divergent.

As each team graded at least three other teams, did the teams with better feedback come up with results that were more similar than the teams with worse feedback? The answer was no – the results of both groups were again equally divergent.

In other words, no consensus emerged with increasing statistical qualifications nor with perception of quality. If this study is representative of statistical analyses in general, then there are many different statistical analysis approaches that can be taken that could be judged highly by other statisticians even though those same statisticians may then use a different approach themselves.

Tightening Research Standards

In the past, researchers could take a dataset from a randomised controlled trial and subject it to many different analytical approaches until one of them yielded a publishable result. This so-called p-hacking – trying to get a p-value (probability-value) below 0.05 which is what is often referred to as a statistically significant result, approach struck many scientists as wrong and open to manipulation.

The response has been to demand pre-registration of scientific trials and to demand that the analytical approach be determined before the data is collected in order to stop this method shopping or, as others named it *"torturing the data until it confessed"*.(502)

That may not even work if there was a universally accepted best approach. If there are many equally good approaches leading to many different outcomes, then pre-registering scientific trials will not improve the quality of the results. It, if followed in full, which did not happen, would just lead to the publication of fewer results but they will not be of a better quality – it will either be a question of luck for the researchers that they chose a model that yielded publishable results or there may be an element of skill involved in finding the model that is most likely to give the desired result and consequently leads to high marks from fellow scientists.

If there was a universally accepted best approach, which may not even exist, then having to pre-specify your research result, as outlined in more detail later, will simply mean that the activity is not re'search' but re'confirmation' as it is intrinsically impossible to know the result beforehand when the research covers genuinely unknown territory.

In summary, there seem to be many different approaches to analysing a dataset that are acceptable to statisticians, leading to many different results. More highly qualified statisticians do not come to a better agreement in their analytical approaches when one looks at the results of the approaches. There is also no increase in consensus for the outcome of the analysis with rising praise from fellow statisticians for an analytical approach and its execution.

The question then becomes: Well, what is the truth? Are dark-skinned players in bigger danger of getting a red card or not? If we take some sort of average, i.e. do a crude meta-analysis of the 29 results, then the answer is, "Probably yes, they may be getting about 40% more red cards (odds ratio 1.4) than lighter skinned players but this may be due to confounding factors, with one example of such a factor being a possibility that darker-skinned players are asked to commit more fouls by their trainers than other players". However, there is no way of knowing whether this is true.

The above, much hedged sentence is similar to the conclusion of many systematic reviews, Cochrane reviews and meta-analyses. The unspoken part of the conclusion in such reviews is usually "if we had sufficient high-quality evidence, then we would be able to come up with a firm conclusion but, given the limitations of the original research, we could only make this much weaker conclusion". Looking at the above that assumption is wrong. **Lots of "high-quality" evidence can still lead to inconclusive results because that is intrinsic to the process**

of statistical analysis. Also, corrupted "high-quality" evidence is worse than worthless as such evidence corrupts the outcome of any review or meta-analysis.

For cases such as the above red card example, there is a statistical method called bootstrapping that would also give an estimate for the range of the percentage, leading to a statement like: "There is substantial evidence that darker skinned players get 40% more red cards with the most likely range (the 95% confidence interval) being 22% to 60%, hence we recommend ..." where the recommendation may be extra referee training or, for example, a recommendation for panels that decide on further punishments for the red-carded player after the game to take into account that dark-skinned players may, through no reason other than their skin colour, be more likely to receive a red card or that further research is necessary to ascertain whether darker skinned players are more likely to play rough, possibly to impress their peers and the coach or because they are more likely to be used as enforcers on the field and therefore reasons other than skin colour may be responsible for the higher number of red cards and also whether this effect changes over time.

The pharmaceutical industry has in practice as its main purpose to increase shareholder value, as the managers' incentives are aligned more or less directly with the share price, which means that, if lies increase shareholder value more than the truth does, then it is financially desirable for research to be used to disseminate lies, a process which has been well documented in these two and many other books: (60, 91). In fact, there is now what can only be described as an industry of pharma-bashing literature, most of which seems to be of a very low standard.

Examples can be found by searching for books with the word 'pharma' in the title on amazon.com.

Medical research is by definition considered to be about people and their health(503) and the current implementation of medical research has done an amazing job in finding helpful new items of knowledge.

However, evidence-based medicine has conspicuous failures as entire societies are getting more and more obese and every second person is expected to get cancer in their life, which means that despite enormous research efforts, the rate of cancer is not dropping. That rate is not dropping despite the successful initiatives to increase screening for cervical, breast, bowel and prostate cancer and to reduce smoking and binge drinking, which means the expectation for an individual to have cancer in their life is definitely not dropping. Also, evidence-based medicine has major difficulties with patients who have multiple ailments (multiple morbidities or co-morbidities) as it is difficult if not impossible to design trials for such patients(120, 504, 505) and multiple co-morbidities can lead to unwanted interactions between treatments.(506) These are just some examples where evidence-based medical research is unable to stem the tide.

Medical doctors and patients are aware of the deficiencies of evidence-based medicine, which has resulted in more money being spent on non-evidence-based medicine,(507-512) something I find deeply ironic. By overstating its case and controlling and hampering doctors, evidence-based medicine is creating a backlash of increasing use of non-evidence-based treatments and suppressing that backlash may not be the answer.

Are Randomised Controlled Trials Settled Science?

'Settled science' is a vague concept that has been heavily used during COVID-19 to quash statements that go against the prevailing narrative. Here 'settled science' means that there is a broad consensus among researchers with little change to that consensus in recent times. Another definition of 'settled science' may be a situation where the scientific consensus is close to the actual truth of a particular matter and that evaluation is shared by most researchers in that area.

When I presented the above question about randomised controlled trials to statisticians their comments were typically that this is true, or more accurately, undeniable, for observational studies but not for randomised controlled trials. That strikes me as disingenuous as a lot of manipulation still allows such trials to be published in top medical journals as described many times in this book you are now reading, with the c19.org websites(153, 238) showing that, when a particular narrative is required, at times and certainly in recent times only false or heavily manipulated results are published in the most prestigious journals.

Day-to-day examples of such manipulated statistics are:

Not recording the doctor in multicentre trials, only recording the centre, thereby avoiding the need to account for a doctor clustering effect and therefore overstating the measured effect – according to a clinical trial specialist's private communication to me this non-recording is ubiquitous.

Comparing the investigated treatment against a placebo instead of against best existing practice.

When the investigated treatment is compared against an existing remedy, then under- or overdosing the existing treatment or giving it against the manufacturer's instructions, such as timing.

Testing treatments only on healthy and or younger volunteers instead of the actual target market of older patients who already are on multiple interventions (pills or other treatments).

When older people are tested, then only recruiting subjects with no co-morbidities (other ailments) or who take no other relevant medicines.

The unclarity whether a trial needs to be single blind (patient does not know what they get), double blind (patient and doctor) or triple blind (patient, doctor and data analyst). That discussion is usually moot as the patients receiving the investigated treatment can easily be identified by the side effects of the treatments.

Once patients are identified by their treatment, a whole universe of manipulation opens up by selectively diagnosing or not diagnosing one group, treating the two groups differently, dropping patients who do badly in the treatment group, dropping patients who do well in the control group, continuously analysing the trial data and stopping at a favourable point, substituting end points as the trial may go badly for overall mortality but may go well for reduction in an intermediate marker such as cholesterol levels, changing what is measured etc etc.

A science that allows outright and often outrageous manipulation is not settled.

These days medical research results are re-investigated more often than has happened in previous decades, showing a high percentage of them to be false or, at best, to be highly variable. (142, 440, 442, 472) This means that running the same or a very similar trial can and often does lead to a very different result.

These different results are partly a simple consequence of mathematics(513-515) but also, as the variations are bigger than mathematics predicts, seem to be the consequence of manipulating the reported outcome through a wide variety of means. (142, 516-518)

CHAPTER 14

HOW DOES A MEDICAL TRIAL WORK?

Medical Trials Are A Big Subject But Essentially, Most of Them Have the Following Elements:

A number of people receive a treatment, a *"prophylactic, diagnostic or therapeutic procedure"*(503) and the trial assesses whether the treatment has a benefit and whether it causes any harm.

The assessment is done by measuring something, for example lung capacity or cancer tumour size before and after a treatment.

If there is a difference, statistics are used to measure whether the difference could have arisen by chance. If that is <u>unlikely</u> (it is very rare for it to be <u>impossible</u> to have arisen by chance), then a medical professional checks whether that difference makes the treatment important enough to use, the phrase being "whether the finding has clinical significance".

There are so-called observational trials where procedures and events are simply recorded and then there are intervention studies where *"new preventative measures, programmes or treatments that are designed to reduce ill health or promote good health"* are measured.(519)

Observational studies fall into a number of types of study. Their main weakness is that something important may not have been recorded.

They can still be compelling as shown in 1747 when a person tried several different treatments for scurvy with citrus fruits working far better than any of the alternatives.(519) However, it is always possible to have doubt, even in the case of smoking causing lung cancer where observational studies showed the risk of smokers developing lung cancer to be much higher than that of non-smokers. At the time these findings came out, statisticians (most of whom, like the general population, were smoking) pointed out that there may be an unknown second cause associated with smoking causing cancer and hence why they could not be sure that reducing smoking would make a difference.

This reasoning is less far-fetched than it sounds because it is true for coffee consumption and lung cancers. Coffee drinkers clearly have an increased risk of developing lung cancer but reducing or stopping coffee by itself would not reduce the risk of developing lung cancer. Why? The reason is that coffee drinkers are more likely to be smoking, and it is this increase in smoking that causes the extra lung cancers.

Of course, this numbers-driven approach ignores the fact that, if we take measures to reduce the drinking of coffee, then they may also reduce other risky behaviour like smoking or lack of exercise. Interdependencies are difficult for science to handle, and a lot of effort is made to isolate behaviours and treatments to make investigations easier.

Observational studies can have just one patient (a case study) or a few patients only or they can be very large like the Framingham cohort study where 5,209 residents of a suburb of Boston have been observed since 1948 which among other results yielded many findings between lifestyle choices and chronic conditions and the long term effects of chronic conditions such as diabetes.(520-522)

Depending on the type of study, the findings of observational studies are considered more or less reliable. At the bottom are case studies because anything can happen to a single person. However, they are very useful for discovering a new disease, for finding cases where existing drugs work for other ailments, known as repurposing or off-label prescription or to report any unexpected medical outcome for a patient, as some examples.

Next up are ecological studies which attempt to establish a link between the so-called exposure and an outcome (usually a disease). For example, it was found that a correlation (a mathematical connection) exists between a bacterium (helicobacter pylori) and gastric cancer in China(523) and this correlation also existed in other countries while other observational studies disputed this association.(524) Here the association turned out to be true but it could have easily been a coincidence or a similar situation as with coffee and lung cancer above.

If the association was true, then there were bismuth-based antibiotics available to treat gastric ulcers, but it took the discoverers of this treatment years until it was generally accepted, for which the discoverers eventually received the 2005 Nobel Prize for medicine.

Other types of observational studies record lots of details about individuals, comparing individuals with ailments with other individuals that are very similar in demographics but do not have the ailment. They are called case-control studies and cross-sectional studies that fall under the category of "interesting but not conclusive".

An example of a case control study is 50 people with a rare type of cancer. The researchers then try to find 100 other people who are as similar as possible to the cancer patients but who do not have that cancer. They look to see if there are any substantial differences between the two groups. The weakness of these two types of studies is that they look at people who already have the disease or outcome, which means they look at a very select group of people and any conclusions may simply not hold for the general population.

Another type of observational study, such as the Framingham study, has a high reputation, but it is very expensive: Hundreds, thousands or even hundreds of thousands of people are recruited and many types of measurements are taken. Then, these people are observed, sometimes over decades, and how those who develop a particular disease or outcome differ from the rest of the population is recorded. For example, the Framingham study mentioned above showed that smoking, high cholesterol levels, high blood pressure, obesity and lack of physical activity are associated with heart disease.

However, there is no relatively cheap observational study with a high reputation which is considered to be acceptable as there is another type of study that does have a high reputation and is relatively cheap compared to the Framingham study: The intervention study and in particular, the randomised controlled trial.

An intervention study recruits a number of participants and gives them a treatment while measuring them a number of times. The purpose is to see if there are any differences between the measurements.

Intervention studies without a control group are not considered reliable because any improvement recorded could be down to a host of reasons not connected to the intervention. An example is that people often get better simply by being treated, which is one of the aspects of the placebo effect.

Hence an intervention trial, where you divide the patients into two or more groups and treat these groups as close to similar as possible so that all have the same placebo effect for example, gives you more certainty that there is a genuine difference between the different treatments.

There is still one problem. We may end up with very unbalanced groups. An obvious example is one group being mostly women and another group mostly men, though the difference may not be at all obvious at times, such as more people suffering from depression in one of the groups compared to another.

The answer to this dilemma is to allocate the patients randomly to each group. We then do not need to know whether a person is depressed or not, the randomisation makes it more likely that roughly equal numbers of, for example, people with depression or men and women end up in each group. The beauty of this approach is that we do not need to know the depression status of the participants, the randomisation simply allocates them in roughly equal numbers to each group. But there is a chance that even with randomisation we can end up with very imbalanced groups, similar to throwing a dice and getting a sequence of '5' and '6', though there are ways to deal with this if we know what we are looking for:

We can stratify the groups, for example make sure that equal numbers of men in women are in each but if we are not aware of a patient characteristic that could be important, like depression status, then randomisation is our best shot at getting roughly equal groups and we have to accept that at times we will be unlucky. The bigger the two groups, the less likely will it be that there are major imbalances as any medical statistics textbook will advise.

The benefits of randomisation give a much higher level of credibility to a randomised controlled trial. Mathematically, the randomisation makes it possible to combine the results of multiple trials through what is called meta-analysis. The results of meta-analyses are considered even more reliable than a single randomised controlled trial.

Randomised controlled trials

Hence and following on from the above, randomised controlled trials and meta-analyses, which combine the results from multiple trials, reign supreme as the most reliable form of trial(521, 522)

The question arises here whether randomised clinical trials, even if they are of higher evidentiary quality than observational and other studies, are really the arbiters of truth or gold standard(525, 526) that they are made out to be.

Randomised controlled trials have a few issues. The word 'controlled' indicates that the intervention is compared to a control treatment, which may for example be the standard treatment or a placebo. The first issue is that substantially similar or even identical trials come up with quite different results(527, 528) and as any meta-analysis of multiple trials shows that many published results, even for these randomised controlled trials, are so contradictory that a proportion of them have to be false. There are simply too many possibilities to get it deliberately or inadvertently wrong when conducting such a trial, making the trial and therefore the outcome suspect or invalid.

Another completely separate but very interesting point is that the results of trials are very similar, regardless of whether people are being randomly allocated or are allocated by their own preferences.(529)

This is a very unexpected result as, when you learn about running clinical trials, you hear lots of stories where doctors 'gamed' the random allocation to give their needier patients the treatment that the doctors considered the better treatment (whether that was the tested treatment or the control treatment). The new insight here is that if the patient made the choice whether to have the tested or the control treatment, the patients in this particular research setting allocated themselves just as effectively across the two treatments as randomisation would have done.

While, if doctors allocate patients to one of the two treatments, it is only one or two people making such a decision and then you get, for example, all the sicker patients in one group and the healthier patients in the other group as the doctor considered the first group was receiving the better treatment. In that case any comparison between the treatments becomes useless because systematically different populations are being treated. This systematic difference did not happen in the above research. The attraction of patients allocating themselves is that these patients are more motivated to stay with the trial as trial dropouts can be a major problem in clinical trials as they make statistical evaluation of the results harder or impossible.

If the preference comes from the patient, randomisation may not be needed. If the preference comes from the organiser, randomisation will most likely be needed.

The disadvantage of that approach is that patients choosing their own treatment is not widely accepted as a valid method of allocation.

Randomisation takes away the choice of intervention from the doctor. It is understandable if that would make doctors uncomfortable when participating in randomised controlled trials as that could mean that patients are, in the doctor's opinion being assigned to the wrong treatment for that particular patient. In other words, the randomisation may actually cause harm to the patient by interfering with the judgment of the doctor at least in some cases.

The main purpose of randomisation therefore may be less for statistical reasons, as persuasive as these may be, but to reduce a source of bias from the organisers or health professionals of a trial.

Highly Variable Results

The below 2005 quote from the paper titled '*Why most published research findings are false*'(142) gives a summary of the ways scientific studies are falsified. The quote uses the expression 'study power', meaning 'statistical power'. Statistical power is bigger if more people are in the trial and if the measured effect is larger. The more power, the better, as higher statistical power increases the probability that a result in a scientific study is a true result, and a lack of a result is due to there being no effect if no corruption is involved:

> '*There is increasing concern that most current published research findings are false. The probability that a research claim is true may depend on study power and bias, the number of other studies on the same question, and, importantly, the ratio of true to no relationships among the relationships probed in each scientific field. In this framework, a research finding is less likely to be true when the studies conducted in a field are smaller; when effect sizes are smaller; when there is a greater number and lesser preselection of tested relationships; where there is greater flexibility in designs, definitions, outcomes, and analytical modes; when there is greater financial and other interest and prejudice; and when more teams are involved in a scientific field in chase of statistical significance. Simulations*

*show that for most study designs and settings, it
is more likely for a research claim to be false than
true. Moreover, for many current scientific fields,
claimed research findings may often be simply
accurate measures of the prevailing bias.'(142)*

Even if the results of research are actually true, there is still
plenty of scope to then misuse the result. A book from Darrell
Huff(518) is freely available on the internet and describes in
engaging detail how research results can be used to lie or mis-
lead. The original book is from 1954.(517). As mentioned, pharmaceutical and medical device companies are also masters at
bending the scientific process to their will.(60, 91)

Inherent Limitations of the Scientific Discourse

In a speech in 2015 the Economics Nobel prize winner George
Akerlof, while introducing his book *Phishing for Phools*,(490)
co-written with his fellow Nobel laureate Robert Shiller, had
the below to say about what can and cannot be published in
economic science journals and I expect this applies to medical
science journals as well:

*"So this book is going to explore the following
notion; the notion that markets deceive us and
manipulate us. So we have a name for this, we call
this Phishing for Phools. Now all economists know
this. Everybody here in this room knows this, but
that leads to the second very general motivation
[for writing this book].*

The rule of what can and cannot be published in Economics leaves holes. There's some perfectly valid and important things to say, but there's no way to say them that would be acceptable in any economic journal.

For example, quite a few economists, maybe quite a few in this room, thought that financial derivatives would lead to the current crisis. But economists could not figure out, we could not figure out a way to express these views in the form of a paper. So, I believe, that Phishing for Phools is one of those holes in Economics because we all know it, because everybody in this room knows it, it cannot be published.

But because it cannot be published in journal form, then it gets ignored. And because it was ignored, we had the financial crisis and the financial crisis is the central event in the economic history of our time."

The same applies in medical science. Deception or bias, whether conscious or unconscious, is rife in research, leading to poor quality and misleading outcomes. The methods, and the scientific method when applied, are then nevertheless defended as the Only True Way, as the alternatives have all shown major weaknesses as well.

In other words, it is a debate about procedures and neither a debate about truth nor a debate about how research can actually benefit people on a population basis. It is like arguing who had right of way in a nasty car accident when the key purpose is to reduce accidents regardless of who is right and to protect people if an accident happens. Who is responsible pales against these aims unless there was recklessness or intent to cause the accident.

Research should be discerning what is truth and what helps population health as much higher priorities and how to do research as a clear third as research procedures cannot stop intent. I suspect research papers would change dramatically if they needed to answer those two questions rather than just describing what knowledge has been added. Investigating whether there is a procedure that can to a degree automatically discern how much existing research papers discovered a true result and how much a research paper has supported improving population health might be worthwhile and artificial intelligence may be able to assist here.

An initial start could be creating an artificial intelligence model that analyses all, most or many research papers on subjects whether there is consensus or two or more camps and the characteristics of each camp. Further, such a tool may discern how much the results are manipulated, how many expected results are missing and how much the published results needed to be nudged to come to the correct conclusion – provided the AI tool itself is not corrupted as has been happening with major current AI models from Open AI (ChatGPT) and Google (Gemini).

Also, such a tool, if not corrupted, may be able to discern when the prestigiousness of the journal where the result is published is positively or negatively associated with any truthfulness, the positive- or negativeness varying by subject, with COVID-19 a prominent example where the more prestigious the journal, the less reliable the result as shown here as substantiated by the very thorough and continuously updated systematic reviews on c19ivm.org and its sister websites and by Dr Pierre Kory.(468, 530, 531)

What is missing in the application of the research method is a humility that acknowledges that all mind-driven ways to investigate complex systems like the human body or the human mind itself are of poor quality. The mind cannot discern truth, it can only discern logical inconsistencies and recall what it has learned in the past, hence the seemingly strange way that statistics tests hypotheses by specifying the opposite of what the statistician is looking for (the null hypothesis) and then testing, given the data is available, how unlikely the null hypothesis is.

Statistics does not test whether something is true, statistics tests how unlikely the opposite is.

As the mind can only discern inconsistencies and not truth, then, if we are able to sufficiently hide inconsistencies from the minds of our fellow scientists, we can publish anything, regardless of how true it really is. And people do and I am amazed how obvious those lies can be and are still accepted.

Hiding inconsistencies is especially easy when we confirm the prevalent opinion and as long as our methods seem unimpeachable. I have referred several times in this book to Ioannidis' essay listing why most published research findings are false(142) and further, derivative publications.(398, 439-443, 472, 513, 532) That 2005 paper has been downloaded many times but research findings have not become more reliable since.

Evidence-based Medicine: There Is No Truth, There Are Only Rules

The mind cannot discern truth – hypothesis testing

As just mentioned, one of the big surprises when learning statistics is that statistics does not directly decide whether something is likely to be true or not:

If I want to know whether orange juice is good for the treatment of eczema, then I look at the opposite assumption 'orange juice makes no difference to the treatment of eczema', which is called the null hypothesis.

I then look at my dataset and ask, 'how likely is it, that this dataset would happen if the null hypothesis were true', hoping that it is very unlikely, though many statisticians in my experience would dispute that I am engaged in 'hoping' here as I am meant to be a dispassionate researcher, an ideal that is honoured in its breach. If the dataset is unlikely enough, I can then write, 'there is sufficient/strong/substantial evidence that orange juice is beneficial (or harmful) for the treatment of eczema'.

This convoluted approach, which takes some time to understand, uses the ability of the mind to discern inconsistencies as our dataset is inconsistent with 'orange juice makes no difference to the treatment of eczema'. We then describe this inconsistency as 'statistically significant' or, as many statisticians prefer, 'there is poor / good / strong evidence for the fact that ...'

This inconsistency is expressed most commonly in what is called the p-value, which gives the percentage of times such a dataset would arise if the null hypothesis was true.

If there was a 1-in-8 chance such a dataset would arise, then the p-value would be $\frac{1}{8}$ or 0.125. Typically, a threshold of 1-in-20 (p=0.05) is assumed to be statistically significant, i.e. confirming our initial hypothesis – in this case that orange juice is suitable in the treatment of eczema.

There are many ways to improve this naive usage of p-values, but the essence of proving an inconsistency with the opposite of what we are trying to prove remains and one of the main underlying problems is that as a researcher, it very often matters a lot whether the dataset is consistent or inconsistent with the null hypothesis.(533)

Treatment of scientific error

As scientific research is a complicated activity and prone to bias, errors are common. How good is science at fixing errors, once they are identified?

Scientific research has methods for correcting errors, but they do not work very well

"Mistakes in peer-reviewed papers are easy to find but hard to fix", report David B. Allison and colleagues.(534)

Errors in published scientific research can be corrected by pub-lishing a correction of a scientific paper or by withdrawing it. Both methods are highly embarrassing for the author and for the publisher, hence there is a lot of real-world resistance to these two approaches. This is reinforced by finger-pointing and judgmental organisations such as Retraction Watch(535) that do not discern between fraud-related retractions, retractions that are enforced for political motives and retractions that are due to error or retractions that were done in co-operation or against the will of the authors.(536) Retraction Watch has the laudable aim of making it more accessible for researchers to know whether a paper has been retracted as, for example, the citation manager Endnote marks such papers in a researcher's Endnote library but an important outcome of Retraction Watch is that falsely retracted papers get treated just as badly as sci-entific papers retracted because of fraud, which seems to be the most common reason for retractions as scientific outright fraud may be quite prevalent.(136, 137, 537)

It is difficult to eradicate an often-repeated quote, which means a quote that has been cited many times, even if everybody, in-cluding the original author, agree that this truism or quote should be withdrawn, as outlined in a light-hearted article.(538)

The problem is that when we have made up our mind about something, even or especially our collective mind, we become quite blind to seeing even obvious inconsistencies, making the correction of many errors that much harder.

It is made still harder by the tactics employed by people with an agenda, especially if that agenda is to defend the status quo, including suing the messenger such as the ultra-careful Data

Colada blog where three researchers highlight suspected fraud by medical researchers.(136-138, 537) The Data Colada members are interviewed by one of the Freakonomics authors in their podcast.(539)

Another issue may be that fraud is considered to be extremely rare according to prevailing opinion,(540) with only 1 in 5,000 papers or 0.018% considered to be fraudulent.

Why the Proposed Fixes to the Research Issues Will Not Work

There are two developments in medical statistics that reinforce each other:

As a consequence of the disappointing results of most published research findings being false, there is a constant attempt to tighten the standards of scientific reporting like CONSORT 2010. (187) These increased standards do not seem to be designed with anywhere near sufficient cost considerations, making research more and more time consuming and more and more expensive to run.(541, 542)

As a result, we have more and more costly research in medical science that leads to fewer and fewer accepted results.

It would be difficult to imagine a worse outcome for medical research and humanity at large.

The number of published research results keeps rising – but is the number of useful and applicable results rising? If we get more and more useful medical research, then why do we have an obesity epidemic(543) and a rise in many other negative health indicators?

Because medical research primarily concerns itself with procedures, i.e. treatments and causes of disease, not with the well-being of the population,(503) one of the most lucrative outcomes of medical research is the management but not the elimination of chronic diseases. Clearly, medical research needs to concern itself with procedures and causes of disease, but it needs to do so for a purpose. If that purpose is not given its due regard, it is too easy to ignore and concentrate on the means and tools only, which then opens the door to manipulation.

The scientific community is therefore attempting to raise the reliability of the reporting individual research results instead of focussing on the well-being of the population with little regard to the cost in time and money of increasing that reliability.

It is easy to establish that there is large scale waste in medical research(398, 439, 440, 443, 472, 532, 544) but the question is not investigated whether eliminating or reducing waste is the most efficient approach, evaluated by the number of new, useful research findings becoming known per dollar spent.

The consequences of high research costs are numerous:

Raising the cost of research raises the stakes for each individual trial, creating stronger and stronger incentives to come up with a result and stronger and stronger disincentives to do research where the outcome is uncertain or even unknown.

Raising the cost of research by trying to live up to an idealised standard means that many trials do not go ahead, as

- potential trials fail a cost-benefit analysis, "*even if the hypothesis is true, it is not worth spending the time and money on it*" and researchers stick to hypotheses that are more likely to lead to a result as only 17% to 21%(545) of research applications get funded. If anecdotal evidence is true, then about 10% of all research applications are obvious funding candidates while a further 60% are 'fundable' but each one of these 60% only has a 1 in 6 to 1 in 9 chance of being funded. This is not a recipe for funding speculative research as there will be more worthy, less speculative applications to be funded. In addition, streamlining research applications does not work(546);
- the interests of those who finance medical trials become more and more important as larger and larger amounts of money are needed for each trial to adhere to the more and more onerous reporting requirements as outlined in the various CONSORT statements;
- findings of harm from lucrative practices and pharmaceuticals are not responded to in time:
  - a pharmaceutical gets wrongly approved by chance or through manipulation of the research and corrective action is delayed (Posicor, Vioxx).(403-405) The story of Vioxx is well told in chapter six of Phishing for Phools;(490)
  - business uses science to find lucrative but ultimately harmful new products and science is

> too slow to respond, often lagging by decades, to show the harm as it is too expensive and time consuming to prove that harm. Examples: Selling cheap food with an addictive mixture of salt, sugar and fat.(126)

The situation is even more stark when we consider that reliable research results are a far inferior marker or outcome than improved population health. Population health can be strongly improved through preventative medicine, lifestyle changes, re-purposing existing out-of-patent drugs and costs can be heavily reduced by using more generic medicines and by emphasising primary care.

Research results that are acceptable as reliable are very important for those whose compounds are being researched, i.e. pharmaceutical companies, as their very substantial financial well-being depends on results to be considered reliable, but for population health reliable research results are of much more minor significance.

So why the emphasis on a less important marker, research results that are considered reliable, than population health?

There is no money in the other measures, they massively reduce costs but there is no sufficient public demand and hence no demand by politicians and regulators to stop all but the worst excesses.

How bad does it need to get? Will we need to destroy our health and bankrupt the systems before we wake up and start taking responsibility for our health and the global corruption?

Pre-registration of scientific trials

When a scientific trial happens that is not steered towards a particular outcome, then the requirements can be so stringent that it makes little sense to have sponsored such a trial in the first place as the chance of reporting a result is so low. An example is the requirement to pre-register certain clinical trials in the United States with clinicaltrials.gov(547) and 'investigators were required to register their primary and secondary outcome variables' which is considered 'important because it eliminates the possibility of selecting for reporting an outcome among many different measures included in the study'. In other words, researchers needed to commit themselves to what the outcome of the trial was before they started the trial and could not cherry pick a result afterwards.

That approach is the opposite of the 'search' in the word 'research' as such research confirms what is known and makes it much more difficult to 'search' for the unknown. If you have to say ahead of your research what you expect to be the type of outcome you are 'researching', you are not engaging in re'search' you are engaging in confirmation or in making sure the result is what is desired by the sponsor.

This pre-specifying requirement makes sense from one point of view as a clinical trial can yield a large number of measurements and, even when there is no underlying effect, purely by chance a proportion of them can show an effect. This process of looking for effects is called p-hacking. On the other hand, what if a true effect was measured that was worth reporting? Is it really sufficient to say that the higher reliability (which is low anyway) is worth the suppression of potentially valuable

findings? Clearly there are trade-offs here but a simple denial of the right to publish such findings may have worse consequences than more unreliable research findings.

A further problem with such an absolutist stance of pre-registering primary and secondary outcome variables is if a
non-prespecified outcome variable shows a very strong result, technically a result with a very low p-value. Such a result
is quite likely to be of interest to the scientific and medical
community but, according to the intent of pre-registering,
should not be worth publishing. In practice, scientific publishers are more lenient than that but why create this conflict
in the first place?

Lately I have heard that it is possible at times to publish such
unpredicted results, provided they are sufficiently strong and
that seems to be a workable compromise – commit before the
trial to what you are looking for but also have the possibility
to report the unexpected.

Why may pre-registering trials be less than optimal? For the
answer we can look at what happened next, once research trials
needed to be pre-registered: Among large cardiovascular trials,
the percentage of those reporting a result dropped from 57%
(17 of 30) before 2000 when trials did not need to be pre-registered to 8% (2 of 25) once trials had to be pre-registered.(541)

An 8% success rate may be too low a percentage for any sponsor.
Hence, ignoring the financial consequences of your requirements
for research trials, requirements that are now often enforced
by ethics panels when scrutinising research proposals, ignoring
the financial consequences may have worse effects – no trials

or trials where there is a thumb on the scale – than being less strict with these research requirements.

Research on procedures and diseases vs research on the health of the patient

There is also something wrong with medical research as practised today which is more fundamental and far reaching:

Medical research is defined as research on procedures and diseases(503) instead of research on the health of the patient. The former is mathematically and conceptually easier to deal with but if you concentrate on only one part of the whole, the intervention, you are unlikely to achieve the optimal outcome for the whole. This is also a reinterpretation of the word "medical: which is defined in the Oxford English Dictionary(482) as *"Pertaining or related to the healing art or its professors"*. In other words, medical research is about healing – animals and people and, since medicine is an art, perhaps medical research should also be an art in addition to being scientifically rigorous.

By making medical research about procedures and diseases, the fact that 'medical' is about healing (of people) is missed and the emphasis is exclusively on some important aspects of healing (procedures and dealing with diseases) but in the process the whole is missed.

We can see the result in ignoring the 'art' part of medicine with our high-cost medical system having a poorer and poorer population health outcome.

It may be possible that most ills of current medical practice can be traced back to this choice.

One of the strongest proponents of evidence-based medicine, John Ioannidis, wrote in a 2016 essay(439) about the issues of evidence-based medicine (EBM):

> *"As EBM became more influential, it was also hijacked to serve agendas different from what it originally aimed for. Influential randomized trials are largely done by and for the benefit of the industry. Meta-analyses and guidelines have become a factory, mostly also serving vested interests. National and federal research funds are funneled almost exclusively to research with little relevance to health outcomes. We have supported the growth of principal investigators who excel primarily as managers absorbing more money. Diagnosis and prognosis research and efforts to individualize treatment have fueled recurrent spurious promises. Risk factor epidemiology has excelled in salami-sliced data-dredged articles with gift authorship and has become adept to dictating policy from spurious evidence. Under market pressure, clinical medicine has been transformed to finance-based medicine. In many places, medicine and health care are wasting societal resources and becoming a threat to human well-being. Science denialism and quacks are also flourishing and leading more people astray in their life choices, including health."*

It makes sense that quacks are flourishing when science allows itself to be so easily subverted in its purpose – improving population health. On the other hand, when the regulated part of medicine fails in its purpose, there is either stagnation or the unregulated part of medicine, which, as it is unregulated, is more dangerous for the patients to participate in, is then an oft-used alternative.

Later in the essay, Ioannidis puts it even more strongly:

"Now that EBM and its major tools, randomized trials and meta-analyses, have become highly respected, the EBM movement has been hijacked. Even its proponents suspect that something is wrong. The industry runs a large share of the most influential randomized trials. They do them very well, they score better on 'quality' checklists, and they are more prompt than nonindustry trials to post or publish results. It is just that they often ask the wrong questions with the wrong short-term surrogate outcomes, the wrong analyses, the wrong criteria for success (e.g., large margins for noninferiority), and the wrong inferences, but who cares about these minor glitches? The industry is also sponsoring a large number of meta-analyses currently. Again, they get their desirable conclusions. ...

Of course, those who are the most successful in grantmanship include many superb scientists. However, they also include a large share (in many places, the majority) of the most aggressive, take-all, calculating managers. These are all very smart people, and they are also acting in self-defense: trying to protect their research fiefdoms in uncertain times. But often I wonder: what monsters have we generated through selection of the fittest! We are cheering people to learn how to absorb money, how to get the best PR to inflate their work, how to become more bombastic and least self-critical. These are our science heroes of the 21st century. ...

However, with 20% of GDP [in the United States] being spent on health and health care so inefficiently, with such limited evidence or with conflicted evidence, medicine and health care can become a major threat to health and well-being. ...

The GDP devoted to health care is increasing, spurious trials, and even more spurious meta-analyses are published at a geometrically increasing pace, conflicted guidelines are more influential than ever, spurious risk factors are alive and well, quacks have become even more obnoxious, and approximately 85% of biomedical research is wasted."

The above is a description of the consequences of evidence-based medicine. What surprises me is that Professor Ioannidis does not consider these issues as being intrinsic to evidence-based medicine. If you substitute a quest for truth with a quest to fulfil rules, would you expect any other outcome? Rules are brilliantly followed. Truth? Population health? Well, ...

If you practise evidence-based medicine, these are the consequences and the cure of these consequences, like pre-registration of trials, is worse than the disease itself as tightening the
reporting of research standards increases the costs of research,
reinforcing the above consequences.

Why would you expect to get a better result from practising
evidence-based medicine by "focusing on ideas, rigorous methods, strong mathematics and statistics"?(439) Why would this
lead to better health outcomes? None of these foci eliminate
the distorting influence of intents and incentives.

An example has been the futility of attempts to deal with the
basic fact that many medical trials do not have enough participants which scientifically expressed means that they lack
statistical power, and their results may have arisen by chance
rather than because there is a true, underlying effect.

A recent paper(548) lists the decade-long attempts to improve
statistical power and stop misusing p-values (roughly, a measure of how likely it is that the researcher has a result on their
hand) and then goes further by modelling the various influences on the quality of research trials. All the models that he
used ended up with researchers doing best who produced the
poorest quality but the highest quantity of results.

Models always only show part of the real world and the models Smaldino and McElreath(548) used are clearly incomplete
but it is interesting that, for example, spending much effort on
replicating medical trials makes little difference to the pes-
simistic outcomes of their models. In other words, according
to these models, the scientific method as currently applied

leads to disaster (large volumes of completely untrustworthy results) and the remedies currently used are not sufficient. Perhaps we are already quite far down this road to disaster.

Smaldino and McElreath's conclusion is quite clear:

> "Whenever quantitative metrics are used as proxies to evaluate and reward scientists, those metrics become open to exploitation if it is easier to do so than to directly improve the quality of research. ... Boiling down an individual's output to simple, objective metrics, such as number of publications or journal impacts, entails considerable savings in terms of time, energy and ambiguity. Unfortunately, the long-term costs of using simple quantitative metrics to assess researcher merit are likely to be quite great."(ibid.)

One question arises:

If there are this many issues with medical research, could it be that there is something very basic that is wrong with medical research?

The answer is yes, there is something very basic that is wrong with medical research.

Evidence and Truth

If we look at the scientific method, which is the way the 'evidence' in evidence-based medicine is gathered, the following points about what is considered to be truth come to mind:

> In the Middle Ages many people in Europe only accepted something as true if it was in the Bible. Today, little seems to have changed as many people that only accept something as true if it is based on scientific evidence, are only considering evidence-based medicine and are ignoring expert consensus medicine.

A vocal group among those who only accept scientific evidence as truth are, surprisingly, referred to as 'skeptics' even though their thinking is based on a particularly narrow foundation and, by implication, their thinking considers truth to be less important than their personal opinion of what truth is. In other words, a skeptic knows they are bigger than truth as they decide what they accept as truth.

The volume of what is accepted as true has increased since the Middle Ages but the mindset has not changed – we put a condition on truth by only accepting a statement as true, if ... and the 'if ...' here is not 'if it is true' but 'if there is sufficient scientific evidence, evidence which is rule based, therefore flawed and open to manipulation'.

This approach is preposterous. Truth is truth, regardless of what shape it appears in.

Besides, this limiting mindset is not working. In medicine, evidence-based medicine is based on published research findings, but to repeat, **most published research findings are false** as John Ioannidis' essay, the most downloaded scientific publication ever, with more than one million downloads, on a big scientific database called PLOS1, reveals in its title.(142, 549)

What happens when a system of knowledge where *"most published research results are false"*, i.e. where most of its knowledge is false, becomes dominant?

The fact that there is a process of sifting and evaluation between research results and eventual clinical practice may improve matters (though this approach is again manipulated as clinical guidelines are often written by industry sponsored experts) but if the foundation is too flawed, no amount of sifting and evaluation will improve the quality of evidence-based medicine beyond a certain point.

Tightening Research Standards – *Are We Shooting Ourselves In The Foot?*

These additional rules that are the outcome of tightened research standards make research much more expensive, raising the stakes for individual undertakings as many research results do not conform to the rules.(541) But despite the additional rules and hurdles that research projects have to overcome there is surprisingly no reduction in published research findings from the worldwide around $260 billion that are spent annually on biomedical research(550) or even trillions.(551)

As it gets increasingly difficult and expensive to do research with the plethora of new rules, researchers switch away from more risky, basic research and from the United States to other nations(552) and generate more scientific publications through a method called 'salami slicing', where scientists publish additional papers by splitting up the content into multiple papers in order to advance their career.(553)

In other words, instead of more useful medical research findings we get more publications as financial and career considerations loom large for many researchers. As one outside commentator remarked:

> *"Improving science by being better at evidence-based results is an utter illusion, for man always affects any result by the intention they have before undertaking the task. This simply means that the scientist and or the researchers are, and will be influencing the results, ... the intention behind the quest will manifest itself in some way, shape or form, and hence, the influence and or manipulation is – inevitable." page 303(554)*

As an aside, many researchers in non-medical research manage to ignore those standards and still get published as shown by the fact that in behavioural science research results from studies with too few participants, studies with insufficient statistical power, to use the technical term, have continually been published over the last 60 years.(548)

All these efforts at tightening research standards, which in practice make research more difficult and expensive, are happening despite some apparent and very large gaps in our knowledge as discussed further on.

We end up with higher and higher costs, less and less new knowledge and understanding plus an overwhelming volume of research output that cannot be trusted and further rules and regulations in reaction to that output.

This deepens the similarities to the Middle Ages where the costs of rituals went up and up as the church acquired more and more wealth(555), the practitioners (priests) became more and more rigid in their adherence to rules,(556, pg 344) the church used up more and more resources by owning more and more land, the primary source of wealth at the time, while providing fewer and fewer additional benefits for a population that was often starving.(557, 558)

Just like in the Middle Ages, where the statement "there are truths in the bible" was turned into "only what is in the bible is true", we now have movements that are turning around the statement "scientific research discovers truths" into "only what is discovered through scientific research can be accepted as true".

An example is the Australian organisation "Friends of Science in Medicine" that, in its principles "*welcome(s) research into traditional and herbal remedies*", though seemingly no other complementary remedies, and states that "*Research into all CAM [so-called Complementary and Alternative Medicine] interventions is a valid role for universities*"(559) while in practice pursuing a very different agenda(560-563) which appears to be to shut down all research into non-allopathic medical practices except for the investigation of traditional medicine.

In the United States, between 28% and 40% of the population believe that the Bible is literally true, is the actual word of God, including 15% of college (university) graduates.(564)

Would it be possible to find a similarly exclusive mindset amongst practising scientists, one that considers the scientific method to be the one and only fountain of truth?

To prove that this fountain is the only true source would require the impossible – proving a negative that *"there is no other way to access truth"*, hence this attitude seems indistinguishable from a myriad of other faith-based statements.

Are There Alternatives To Scientific Research?

It is easy to beat up on science, but things are generally worse everywhere else. There is an enormous volume of falsities, fallacies, misunderstandings and outright lies outside science as shown here(565) and in chapter 4 of this book: (566). In addition, there are also many statements of various sophistication that claim to be scientific, without adhering to scientific standards, that are clearly false, misleading and harmful.(ibid., chapter 9)

It therefore makes sense to rely to a much higher degree on scientific research findings than on statements that come from any other source, but it is a medieval approach to exclude all statements from other sources without proper scrutiny of those statements.

We do need to be aware that scientific research findings are themselves often false, that the sheer volume comes at a significant cost and that the value in useful research findings, those that help people in their lives per dollar spent on scientific research, appears to be going down.(567)

In addition, scientific research still works with the implied assumption that a published research finding should be true. As described earlier, this assumption is not shared by insiders with statistical knowledge who are very sceptical, but it is true for the way scientific results are presented in the press, which includes the many press releases by academic institutions.(568-571) The surprising finding, especially of the latter three referenced papers, is that exaggerated or false claims attributed to scientific trials in the press rarely seem to originate with the journalists but that a minority of the claims were made by the authors themselves in their papers with the majority originating from the press releases of the institutions linked to these researchers. Presumably the researchers had a more or less simple choice between amending the text of the press releases prior to publication of these exaggerated claims and not amending it, which means that they may not have made the claims themselves but allowed them to be made on their behalf and in the name of their research.

There may also be a distinction between journalists who specialise in science and those with no training in science who are able to write blatant untruths about a subject for many years without ever correcting themselves, though very few, if any journalists seem to be prepared to go against the prevailing narrative.

Pharmaceutical companies have made it an art form to provide rule conforming randomised controlled trials that hand favourable results to the products of these companies. Examples are cancer drugs that passed the FDA's scrutiny turn out to have an effect that is indistinguishable from the placebo effect or much more expensive new remedies are no better than existing ones.(91)

Hence, there are major issues with scientific evidence and many scientists are aware of them while the so-called remedies for these issues regularly make things worse as shown in the next section.

Further Issues with Evidence-based Medicine

The rise of evidence-based medicine is coinciding with a rise in childhood diabetes, asthma, hay fever, food allergies, oesophageal reflux and cancer, coeliac disease, Crohn's disease, ulcerative colitis, autism, eczema and obesity,(572, 573). Dantas blames the overuse of antibiotics, which may be a contributing factor, but there may be other important causes as well.

Interestingly, many of the above conditions have a digestive or an auto-immune component or link.

The point is that, despite constant substantial increases in worldwide healthcare spending, many ailments, illnesses and diseases are getting worse.

The rise of evidence-based medicine may be responsible for the fact that these ailments are not impacting us more than they already are. It is also possible that evidence-based medicine may have no connection to these changes or lack of change. However, the mindset of evidence-based medicine, which may be interpreted as "no action without evidence", could be responsible for society holding back on many measures that are becoming more and more urgent. An obvious example might be the decreasing quality and increasing addictiveness of our processed food where the manufacturers use scientific methods for their own purposes(126) while evidence-based medicine lags decades behind in its understanding when and how food is addictive and is falling further and further behind the understanding that manufacturers have. On the face of it, it seems plausible that making food more addictive and less nutritious could lead to deteriorating population health, for example through metabolic syndrome(574) or weight gain.

Benefits of Evidence-based Medicine

There are circumstances where evidence-based medicine works.(120, 121) Examples are that it led to substantial reductions in death from heart (cardiovascular) disease and showed that reducing smoking and high blood pressure together with other preventative measures are at least as effective as medical and surgical interventions to reduce incidences and fatalities of heart disease.(575) The very large WHO MONICA study showed that almost 80% of the 27% worldwide reduction in fatalities from heart disease came from fewer incidences of heart disease and only 20% from improved treatments.(576) Reducing population-based risk factors and improving medical and surgical treatments for heart disease are the results of evidence-based practices.

In the same vein countless trials of cancer medications and treatments have improved the survival rate of cancer patients.

Still, by creating a complex set of rules for what is acceptable to be adopted into clinical practice we have ended up with similar problems to those in another area of life: the tax code.

Because not enough priorities are being set, the sheer volume of evidence-based medicine has become overwhelming. As there are now complex rules, wealthy vested interests like the drug and medical devices industries have been able to manipulate the system through a) controlling the reported outcomes of medical trials while conforming to the rules and b) creating more and more diseases; for example, female sexual arousal disorder or male baldness or even so-called pre-disease states like low bone density, all of which have a new treatment or where the treatment preceded the discovery of the disease(120) and through their influence over those who write guidelines.(97-99, 109, 144-146, 577)

Another obvious outcome of introducing a large body of complex rules is the bureaucracy that has been built around medicine which replaces clinical judgment with rules and guidelines. In certain circumstances this is helpful but it breaks down when the patient does not fit within the rules and guidelines, as is the case in the previously mentioned group with multiple issues (multimorbidity), the incidence of which is rapidly rising in ageing populations.(184)

Even in the 1990s there were already many barriers to the implementation of guidelines as this oft-cited study shows.(143)

Medical trials and statistical tools that sift through data to extract evidence are necessarily broad brush and work either exclusively or largely on a population basis. In fact, medical research explicitly tries to exclude individual patients' variations from their trials. Hence, the evidence may be true for the population as a whole, though this is not at all guaranteed, but it may not apply in many individual cases. An experienced doctor may have developed sufficient heuristics that allow him or her to propose to the patient very different remedies to what evidence-based medicine would recommend – and that physician may well be correct as they take the particular individual into account but such a physician is endangering their ability to get professional indemnity insurance and even their license when they do not follow evidence-base practices.

There is currently no evidence I am aware of that compares traditional and evidence-based medical doctors except for an indirect example where survival rates of heart attack patients increase during cardiovascular medical congresses as more junior and hence more evidence-based doctors direct the treatment of these patients.(578) Hence there may be no way of knowing which of these approaches is better.

CHAPTER 15

WHY THE PROPOSED FIXES TO THE RESEARCH ISSUES WILL NOT WORK – A MORE DETAILED LOOK

Science in Crisis – The Reproducibility Crisis

To any medical statistician, this section is wearily familiar, though some or many of the details may be new, but if you are not a medical statistician, the sheer size of the problem is often a surprise.

Pharmaceutical companies have had major problems translating cancer research into medical treatments. In one famous case, Amgen, a pharmaceutical company with over 20,000 employees, tried to reproduce the results from 53 landmark papers but succeeded to do so in only 6 of them.(444) In other words, 89% of all published results could not be reproduced. Amgen found major mistakes in many of these studies and the author in a later paper(579) felt that the poor quality of results was the outcome of basic science being able to get away with poor work because:

> "In part, it is down to the fact that there is no real consequence for investigators or journals. It is also because many busy reviewers (and disappointingly, even co-authors) do not actually read the papers, and because journals are required to fill their pages with simple, complete 'stories'. And because of the apparent failure to recognize authors' competing interests—beyond direct financial interests—that may interfere with their judgement.
>
> Every biologist wants and often needs to get a paper into Nature or Science or Cell, yet the scientific community fails to recognize the perverse incentive this creates. Some of these issues could be readily addressed by publishing only blinded, replicated and appropriately controlled preclinical experiments."

However, note that the author considers that only *"some of these issues"* can be addressed by tightening up the scientific methodology.

Bayer Healthcare in Germany reported in 2011 that in only about 20-25% out of 67 of their projects

> "the relevant published data (was) completely in line with our in-house findings. In almost two-thirds of the projects, there were inconsistencies

between published data and in-house data that either considerably prolonged the duration of the target validation process or, in most cases, resulted in termination of the projects because the evidence that was generated for the therapeutic hypothesis was insufficient to justify further investments into these projects".(397)

Ed Yong, in an article in Nature in 2012, lists many and substantial weaknesses of psychological research:

"Positive results in psychology can behave like rumours: easy to release but hard to dispel. They dominate most journals, which strive to present new, exciting research. Meanwhile, attempts to replicate those studies, especially when the findings are negative, go unpublished, languishing in personal file drawers or circulating in conversations around the water cooler. 'There are some experiments that everyone knows don't replicate, but this knowledge doesn't get into the literature,' says Wagenmakers. The publication barrier can be chilling, he adds. 'I've seen students spending their entire PhD period trying to replicate a phenomenon, failing, and quitting academia because they had nothing to show for their time.'

These problems occur throughout the sciences, but psychology has a number of deeply entrenched cultural norms that exacerbate them. It has become common practice, for example, to tweak experimental designs in ways that practically guarantee positive results. And once positive results are published, few researchers replicate the experiment exactly, instead carrying out 'conceptual replications' that test similar hypotheses using different methods. This practice, say critics, builds a house of cards on potentially shaky foundations."(580)

In the psychological sciences, reproducing 100 studies showed that only 36 of the replicated studies had significant results, though in a further 11 studies the original and the replicated study had statistically consistent results .(581) A statistically consistent result can come about because each statistical finding comes with an uncertainty range (the confidence interval). If two findings are different but their confidence intervals overlap, then they are statistically consistent. Overall, the measured effect of all studies combined dropped by half. Their conclusion:

"A large portion of replications produced weaker evidence for the original findings despite using materials provided by the original authors, review in advance for methodological fidelity, and high statistical power to detect the original effect sizes. Moreover, correlational evidence is consistent with the conclusion that variation in the strength of initial evidence (such as original P value) was more predictive of replication success than variation in the characteristics of the teams conducting the research (such as experience and expertise)."

In other words, the strength of the evidence found was more important than the reputation of the researchers when it came to deciding whether a finding was reproducible or not. Many more details about the abuses of drugs for mental health are found in Peter Gøtzsche's publications.(60-62, 128, 370, 582-588)

Examples of Influence That Can Affect Research

Here are some influences that can affect many different areas of research and many different types of research trials.

Bias is defined as *"the combination of various design, data analysis and presentation factors that tend to produce research findings when they should not be produced"*(142) and by the Oxford English Dictionary as *"A systematic distortion of an expected statistical result due to a factor not allowed for in its derivation; also, a tendency to produce such distortion."*

There are many examples in epidemiology (evidence-based medicine research is simply another way of expressing 'using epidemiological practices in medical research' – they are very similar if not the same). Spurious connections between cause and effect are constantly reported in the press due to great interest in those results. "Computers cause breast cancer" is an easy headline to catch attention.(589) These spurious connections are among the biggest reasons for any decline in the general public's trust in research findings as in many cases, sooner or later, another study with a different if not opposing result gets published.

Another good example is the reporting of research results on alcohol and humans. Here the reporting is highly distorted as findings that are favourable to alcohol consumption find an easy and eager audience while more negative findings receive less coverage. A public consensus at the moment seems to be that regular consumption of red wine reduces the risk of heart disease and that this positive effect outweighs any negative effects, like an increased risk of cancer for example. My reading of the literature is that the research results are inconclusive with a wide range of findings. Statements that alcohol is highly harmful or quite beneficial could both be consistent with the evidence from the current research findings.

Statistical techniques that could routinely be used to bias medical research

One of these statistical techniques is called directed chance – the smaller a trial is, the more likely it is that a result has shown up purely by chance. As results fluctuate this can be magnified by constantly evaluating the trial and stopping it at a convenient moment and when the fluctuation is particularly large and pointing in the desired direction which can then substantially if not conveniently distort the reported result.

Furthermore, so-called outliers tend to be routinely removed from data – for example a recording of human height of 30cm or 300cm. However, a proportion of these, like a human height of 70cm or 230cm, may be a true measurement and will materially affect the result when removed.

Reverse bias is the opposite – true findings are not reported because the researcher does not notice them through mistakes or error in the analysis or because they are inconvenient (side effects of an intervention or treatment for example).

Examples of influence that can steer even a meta-analysis of randomised controlled trials

As previously outlined in detail in Chapter 10, there are a number of different kinds of medical studies with very different levels of credibility in the eyes of medical regulators. The study type with the most credibility is the randomised controlled trial where a treatment gets tested against a control, which can be another treatment or a placebo. That means a randomised controlled trial has at least two groups, the treatment group and the control group and the crucial point is that participants are randomly allocated to either one of them.

The only type of publication with even more credibility is an analysis of multiple randomised controlled trials and sometimes other research evidence, which is called a meta-analysis or systematic review. In a meta-analysis the results of multiple randomised controlled trials are combined and, if done well and if the results of the underlying trials are credible, then the results of the meta-analysis are even more reliable.

Multiple meta-analyses or systematic reviews are typically used to set public policy and to write guidelines on which treatments are recommended, acceptable, have unknown efficacy or are not recommended.

However, the following is a list of issues that can affect a meta-analysis and its constituents, randomised controlled trials – if the underlying trials are all biased in the same way, then the meta-analysis will be equally biased.

This is in addition to the fact that meta-analyses are now being debased through mass-production.(532)

The sponsor of the trial. If the sponsor is expecting a financial return on their investment, then this is a strong, well accepted and increasing influence on any result.(425, 590, 591) If the sponsor does not expect a financial return, there is still the pressure to come up with a result. Even the most patient sponsor of basic research will restructure if insufficient results are forthcoming.

Publication bias. Studies with a result are more likely to be published, especially in prestigious journals. Likewise, studies where the result suits the sponsor's interest are more likely to be published.(148, 162, 220, 271, 413)

In addition, if the **sponsor has strong control over the research process**, for example in commercial in-house research of pharmaceuticals, studies that are not promising can be terminated, not published, their publication delayed, or their findings 'softened' while helpful studies can be continued. The published results can then be far from the truth, with either the positive effect being exaggerated or the true positive effect being no different from the placebo effect. This is shown by the following quote (221):

> *"Over the past 2 decades, the pharmaceutical industry has gained unprecedented control over the evaluation of its own products. Drug companies now finance most clinical research on prescription drugs, and there is mounting evidence that they often skew the research they sponsor to make their*

drugs look better and safer. Two recent articles underscore the problem: one showed that many publications concerning Merck's rofecoxib that were attributed primarily or solely to academic investigators were actually written by Merck employees or medical publishing companies hired by Merck."

And:

"The problem is not so much the sponsorship itself but the terms. Before the 1980s, industry grants to academic institutions to fund studies by faculty members gave investigators total responsibility. The investigator designed the studies, analyzed and interpreted the data, wrote the papers, and decided where and how to report the results. Generally, neither the investigators nor their institutions had other financial connections to sponsoring companies.

In recent years, however, sponsoring companies have become intimately involved in all aspects of research on their products. They often design the studies; perform the analysis; write the papers; and decide whether, when, and in what form to publish the results. In some multicenter trials, authors may not even have access to all their own data."

Personally, I am not sure at all that there is a way to sponsor medical trials without the sponsor's or the researchers' interests being taken into account and thus a conflict of interest inviting all that has been outlined in this book and more.

Evidence-based medicine says that if you follow the rules, your results count as evidence and can therefore be treated as truth. Pharmaceutical companies change the rules by creating conflicts of interest(591) that would have been deemed unacceptable in the past through sheer force of money and otherwise follow the rules, better than non-industry researchers, but the results rather often favour their own products.(148, 162, 220) Their arsenal of incentives for researchers include, for example, consulting and speaking fees, advisory board memberships, fees, employment and research grants. If the results do not favour the sponsor, the trial results may not be published, which is commonly referred to as publication bias.(125, 162)

The most influential medical scientific publications on guidelines tend to be systematic reviews or meta-analyses, especially of multiple randomised controlled trials. Even if conflicts of interests for the original trials are reported, those conflict details are rarely also reported in meta-analyses.(592)

Unsurprisingly, conflicts of interests in other research areas are a problem as well, such as this example from economics.(593)

Another arrangement helpful for the pharmaceutical industry are companies, called contract research organisations with the sole purpose being industry research with networks of physicians who, alongside other possible payments, get paid for providing patients for research trials. One of the strongest levers are industry supported start-ups in which academic or clinical (doctor) researchers have, in some cases, multi-million-dollar stakes. For example, the chairman of the psychiatry department at Stanford University had a $6 million stake in a company that developed a pill for psychotic depression while that same chairman was the principal investigator for a government grant that included researching the value of that very pill. Initially, Stanford University supported the arrangement and only later stopped it when public pressure mounted.(221)

When it comes to influencing the outcome of clinical trials of drugs, pharmaceutical and medical device companies are both subtle and effective about their influence,(162, 220, 594) even in surgery.(426)

With all these difficulties in producing reliable research results, the question arises whether there is something fundamental that is missing or misunderstood in medical research.

And there is, as is shown in the following.

The Purpose of Medical Research Is Procedures and Diseases, Not Human Well-Being

The World Medical Association in its 1952 "Declaration of Helsinki"(503) defined the purpose of medical research as:

> *"The primary purpose of medical research involving human subjects is to improve prophylactic, diagnostic and therapeutic procedures and the understanding of the aetiology and pathogenesis of disease. Even the best proven prophylactic, diagnostic, and therapeutic methods must continuously be challenged through research for their effectiveness, efficiency, accessibility and quality."*

In other words, medical research is about procedures and diseases. The primary purpose of medical research involving human subjects is not improving the well-being of human subjects, even though the word 'medical' is about the 'healing arts'.(482)

It is clearly implied that, by improving procedures and diseases, the well-being of human subjects is improved but **it is not the** primary **purpose of medical research to improve the well-being of human beings.**

This is where we went wrong.

We are more and more concentrating on improving procedures and understanding disease as if they could be considered separately from human beings, but we are not working on improving people's well-being as our primary purpose.

This declaration also refers to human "*subjects*", which is not the same as "people".

We have missed the point that medical research is about improving the well-being of people, i.e. that medical research is about the healing arts. We are only concentrating on certain aspects of improving the well-being of people – on procedures and understanding disease.

Should medical research not be about healing the whole of a person?

As Plato wrote 380 B.C.E.(595):

"That as you ought not to attempt to cure the eyes without the head, or the head without the body, so neither ought you to attempt to cure the body without the soul; and this is the reason why the cure of many diseases is unknown to the physicians of Hellas, because they are ignorant of the whole, which ought to be studied also; for the part can never be well unless the whole is well."

The Limitations of Procedures

Procedures ignore the one who is undertaking the procedure – the medical professional – and, according to the Helsinki Declaration, consider the one who is receiving the procedure – the patient – a subject.

According to the Oxford English Dictionary the definitions of the word "subject" are replete with ideas of a person being controlled or inferior (subjects of a ruler, in law a thing over which a right is exercised or a piece of property, in logic the thing a judgment is made about) with the main medical definition being *"A person who presents for or undergoes a medical or surgical treatment; hence one who is affected with some disease"*.

Ethics

A big part of medical research is ethics. All research on humans is supposed to be vetted by an ethics panel to make sure that the particular kind of research is worth the money, time or physical or mental suffering of the study participants and/ or the researchers.

An ethical review can either be expedited if the impact is minimal and the research subject is not an intervention – for example a review of stored public data – or a full application in all other cases. Full ethics applications also contain a scientific review of the proposed trial and typically take several months during which the study cannot start and any amendments to the study protocol will need to be approved again. In other words, ethics applications make research considerably more time consuming and expensive.

The justification for ethics applications is derived from the perversion of research by Dr Mengele and others in World War II concentration camps out of which the Nuremberg Code(596) was created at the end of the Nazi doctors' trial in 1947.

A full ethical application today has many more components than just the ethical issues. You are asked for a full study protocol rather than just the ethical issues for your research. This is justified with the reasoning that it would be unethical to subject people to a not-fully-considered study and is a typical example how a good idea – treating people who are subject to research ethically – balloons into a large bureaucratic edifice and hand control over research to what may well be unsuitable people.

This makes research more cumbersome and rigid, as making changes becomes more expensive in terms of time and effort and imposes a large barrier to entry as writing a high-quality protocol requires both experienced clinicians and statisticians.

To study the effect of a simple massage treatment, for example, requires a full ethical review as it is an intervention therapy and necessitates a long and detailed study protocol to fulfil the 'ethical' requirements. This is despite massage having been used for thousands of years and millions of people receiving one every day. However, if you want to *research* massage ...

Interestingly, if you have enough political power, you may be able to bypass ethics altogether: If your research is not about humans or is purely analysing public data, you may not need an ethics application. If a scientific journal accepts that your research is about data, not humans, you can go ahead without one.

A particularly blatant misuse of this 'loophole' is a large, 2016 published trial(204) on surgical residents (newly minted surgeons who have to work in hospitals under exploitative conditions for a period of time) where these students and residents either had the normal rules of working no more than 80 (!) hours a week or almost no rules at all about their working hours.

No ethics panel would be likely to accept research on humans that would subject them to the existing regime of 80-hour weeks for surgical residents, let alone an even more onerous one. However, many authors of this study were in powerful administrative positions, so the New England Journal of Medicine, one of the most prestigious publications, allowed the authors to classify the research as 'non-human' as the researchers only analysed the resulting data. Clearly, this is a lie as the residents were, as part of the research, randomly allocated to either of the two regimes, which means that something was done to them, an intervention, which should have involved a full ethical review.

It is a cheap shot to point out one of the many misuses of research, but this particular manipulation is especially blatant and perpetrated by the most senior members of the medical profession and one of the most prestigious journals, so it is quite a remarkable example of the actual corruption in research practices. It may be no surprise that the paper is also riddled with bias, for example: A half way review of the one-year trial was done to evaluate patient safety, but only unexpected mortality was used as a parameter, not something more pertinent like post-surgery complications and the safety of the surgical residents was completely ignored in the study – the half-year review did not mention the well-being or safety of the residents at all.

It is interesting that such a senior group of researchers and clinicians used their power to bypass the ethics process altogether. Was it just a demonstration of their power, a complete disdain of their subjects (surgical residents) or a strong indication that in the assessment of these researchers and clinicians the ethics process had gone overboard so they felt justified in bypassing it altogether, or even simpler, because their study would never have passed ethical scrutiny?

Examples of Meta-Analysis

This example of a meta-analysis is from an article in the British Medical Journal reviewing a number of randomised trials checking whether supplements have an influence on cardiovascular disease. Note in the graph below the differences between the trial results (the squares) among the trials. Some squares are on the left which means they show that using supplements has a favourable influence on cardiovascular disease. Other trials are at or very near the dotted vertical line which means that their result does not favour either supplements or using no supplements. There are no boxes on the right, so there is no evidence that supplements have a negative influence on cardiovascular disease.

Meta Analysis

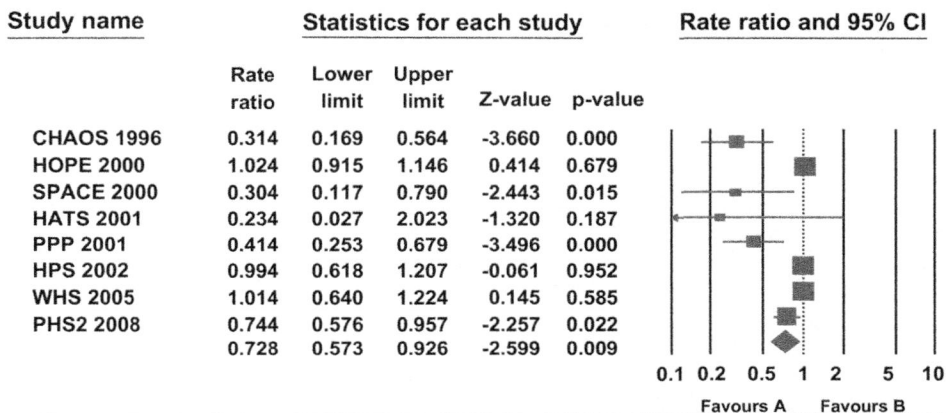

Study name	Statistics for each study					Rate ratio and 95% CI
	Rate ratio	Lower limit	Upper limit	Z-value	p-value	
CHAOS 1996	0.314	0.169	0.564	-3.660	0.000	
HOPE 2000	1.024	0.915	1.146	0.414	0.679	
SPACE 2000	0.304	0.117	0.790	-2.443	0.015	
HATS 2001	0.234	0.027	2.023	-1.320	0.187	
PPP 2001	0.414	0.253	0.679	-3.496	0.000	
HPS 2002	0.994	0.618	1.207	-0.061	0.952	
WHS 2005	1.014	0.640	1.224	0.145	0.585	
PHS2 2008	0.744	0.576	0.957	-2.257	0.022	
	0.728	0.573	0.926	-2.599	0.009	

0.1 0.2 0.5 1 2 5 10

Favours A   Favours B

Meta Analysis

The question for this meta-analysis is whether the overall evidence is supportive of using supplements or is not supportive. Here are the results in graphical form:

Each square is a clinical trial. Such trials tend to go by a name (usually a more-or-less contrived acronym) like CHAOS or HOPE. The size of the square in the graph shows the size of the trial. The horizontal line shows the plausible range of the research results (the 95% confidence interval) – the longer the line, the less informative is the trial. A trial where the horizontal line touches or crosses the dotted vertical line in the middle (labelled '1') is, by itself, inconclusive but its data is still useful in the meta-analysis.

The rhomboid is the combination of the trials.

The horizontal lines coming out of the squares show how certain the result was – the shorter the lines, the better – the horizontal line displays what is called the confidence interval which means that the true result is 95% likely to sit anywhere on the horizontal line, with the centre of the line the most likely place and the ends substantially less likely, but any spot on the line is a possible place for the square. This shows the level of certainty of the result – the shorter the line, the more authoritative the finding becomes. There is also a 5% probability that the true result is to the left or right of the horizontal line.

The size of the square shows the number of participants in the trial: the more participants, the bigger the square.

You may also notice that the bigger squares have shorter horizontal lines – the larger the number of participants, the more 'statistical power' and the less uncertain the result becomes.

The rhombus, a 'square' where all sides have the same length, but the angles need not be 90º as in a square, shows the result if you mathematically combine all the trials.

There are a lot of interesting details in this table.

If the horizontal line of a trial touches the solid vertical line, then the result of that trial was inconclusive. The four big trials (with short arms) are all inconclusive while three of the four small trials show a strong result, leading to the overall result (the rhomboid) being to the left of the vertical line, meaning that supplements seem to help prevent cardiovascular disease.

In this case the mathematics point one way but for an observer, despite the mathematical result, it may be tempting to only conclude that supplements do not seem to cause harm as small trials are less reliable than large trials and the calculations used to combine these results may not take sufficient account of that difference in reliability. Also note the variation in results even though they all test very similar things.

The attraction of randomised controlled trials where multiple trials can be combined for an overall effect in what is called a meta-analysis, is that they are considered to be the best type of trial.

However, it is of note in this case that the three of the four small trials showed a strong effect, and all the big trials did not, so there are really two effects – the small trial effect and the big trial effect with the overall effect mathematically showing that supplements most likely are supportive.

This graph raises the question whether the small trials were manipulated, consciously or unconsciously. It is easier to bias small trials than to bias large trials so this may or may not be the case here. It is also possible that there is a true effect, but the large trials were organised in such a way that this effect was not found, even if there was a true effect. Both are entirely possible, and it is for the reader to decide how they respond to the presented data, but the graph shows one of the problems of meta-analysis: That a number of small trials can give an overall effect even when all large trials show no effect.

Because of the mathematical benefits of randomisation and the ability to combine multiple trials in a mathematically satisfactory way, organisations like the Australian NHMRC (National Health and Medical Research Council) disregard case studies altogether and give far more weight to randomised controlled trials than any other form of research despite their weaknesses.

With statistics, it is possible to find very, very small effects to be statistically significant, provided the dataset is large enough. The question then becomes whether the effect is worth considering in clinical practice. This is determined by deciding whether an effect is large enough to be clinically and not just statistically significant.

The Problems with Randomised Controlled Trials

The insidious point about randomised controlled trials is that there is a seeming solution for almost every individual problem with such trials, but the combined weight of the solutions creates a very high burden on the researchers, making such trials much more expensive for little or no actual gain when one looks at the amount of manipulation that is happening for such trials.

Many clinicians dislike random allocation. They have their own views about the value of the treatment being investigated and want to allocate patients to what they consider the best treatment for them – that is why they studied medicine in the first place. Hence the stories of random allocation being bypassed, if possible, are common.(597) The ostensible solution is to administer the treatment in a way that the clinician does not know which treatment the patient gets and neither does the patient. This is called a double-blind study. A double-blind study where the person analysing the data also does not know what treatments were given to the members of each group is called a 'triple blind study'.

For many procedures / interventions / treatments that level of blinding is physically not possible, so these are at most single blind studies where only the patient is unaware of the treatment. Where it is possible to keep both patients and clinicians from knowing who gets what treatment it is often clear from the 'side effects' who receives which treatment or there could be accidental, slight but detectable differences between the trial and the control treatment. In the latter case the random allocation is not influenced but it may be clear to the staff who gets what treatment, giving rise to a host of possibilities of conscious and unconscious manipulations.

After all, it is striking how well clinical trials paid for by pharmaceutical companies are able to keep to the rules of clinical research and randomised controlled trials, yet come up with a positive result for the companies.(148, 162, 220, 221, 271)

In contrast to today's reality of excellently executed trials that are often wholly unreliable, the Victorian age was an age of very bad research practices but of rapidly increasing true knowledge and medical benefits. Are we moving back towards the stagnation of the Middle Ages with our increasing demand to painstakingly observe more and more rituals? Each individual ritual (research practice) is now justified through evidence, but the consequences of their combined weight are ignored.

A further indication of stagnation is the push to exclude many areas of complementary and alternative practices from university and other sponsored research and the pernicious policy of treating complementary and alternative practices as identical even though their usefulness, intent and clinical practice could be vastly different, as complementary medicine seeks to support and alternative medicine to supplant medicine and medicine is still the most successful way to treat ailments on the planet.(560-563)

Even if, as could be expected from trials held so far, in most cases and possibly in all cases research on alternative treatments will lead to null or negative results, this is still very valuable when it can be shown that certain treatments purely rely on the placebo effect and can then be regarded as such.

Complementary medicine seems to be mostly benign and supportive of the medical treatment it supports such as providing a supportive diet during cancer therapy or to deal with cachexia, i.e. the starvation which is responsible for many cancer deaths.

For alternative medicine, it could be speculated that a treatment may be working by suppressing the symptoms of the underlying complaint with the complaint later returning in perhaps even stronger fashion or with a different set of symptoms, leading to first an improvement and later a worsening of health. On the other hand, many people may get better simply because they are being treated by somebody who cares or they took the initiative to be treated, even if the treatment itself has no effect.

In addition, it may be worth investigating how much a treatment that styles itself as alternative reduces the usage of conventional medicine by the patients choosing that treatment and whether that reduced usage has consequences for the health of these patients. This data may already be available as part of a longitudinal study like the Australian Longitudinal Study of Women's Health and the author has heard anecdotally of such research.

As many patients are overdosed and over-diagnosed(357, 358, 598) and improve when one simply reduces their treatments, one benefit of non-medical treatments in some cases might simply be that they do not harm and their beneficial effect is that they substitute unnecessary or harmful allopathic (medical) treatments.

In conclusion, medical research went wrong right from the start by treating humans as subjects and not as people. We have gone a long way on this wrong track and need to go back to first principles:

What is medical research about?

True medical research is about people and populations, about patients and doctors, the cost of medical treatments and their interactions. All three, patient, doctor and intervention are of equal, vital importance and value.

CHAPTER 16

THE MEDICAL TREATMENT TRIANGLE: THE DOCTOR, THE PATIENT, THE INTERVENTION

There is a comfort in concentrating on the intervention as it means that humans can be more or less ignored when it comes to responsibility for health outcomes, which means being responsible for the healing of humans. These humans are the doctors and the patients themselves in their role of working together on managing, curing or healing the patient.

Hence, for a wider perspective we may consider that worldwide annually in more than a billion(151, 152) medical interactions there are three components:

- The patient
- The doctor
- The treatment

Clearly the patient and the doctor are an important part of this process, but most medical research concentrates on the treatment and either ignores or tries to eliminate the influence of the doctor and exclude the influence of the patient on the result.

This is a ludicrous but a logical consequence of defining medical research on diagnoses and interventions alone.

It is known or at least assumed that healthier doctors have healthier patients.(599, 600) The first reference shows that doctors who themselves follow a supportive primary care practice, which presumably supports their health, are more likely to talk to their patients about this practice. Therefore, physicians who employ at least this one good health practice for themselves make a bigger effort to improve their patients' health in that aspect as well.

Currently science has the widespread belief that it does not know what makes a good doctor and hence does not know how to improve doctors bar increasing their knowledge and experience(601) though more aspects of the above have recently been researched by myself but are not widely known.(64, 65, 68, 192)

Two exceptions are non-peer-reviewed articles which are working papers from the United States National Bureau of Economic Research published in 2014(67) and a particularly well-researched one from 2022(66) already mentioned in Chapter 1 showing that the best Norwegian GPs or family doctors add nine months of life expectancy to their 55+ aged patients compared to the average GP and 18 months compared to the least effective GPs, all this while saving on healthcare costs.

The study also shows that a Norwegian average GP (family doctor) has a 12.2% lower 2-year death rate for their aged 55 and over patients compared to a bottom 5% GP. A top 5% GP also has a 12.2% lower rate than an average GP, adding some $9 million per GP of life expectancy for their patients as a year's life in Norway is valued at $35,000.(66)

My 2023 PhD included published research papers where, with myself as first author, we investigated whether doctors make a difference to patients' physical health even after accounting for all known information such as their demographics and patients' demographics and risk factors. It turned out that doctors make a difference that ranges from the negligible to more than 30% of patients' physical health outcome and the effect often exceeds that of many pharmaceutical therapies.(64, 65)

Further it turned out that there are exceptionally good doctors who consistently perform better than their peers, i.e. they make an even bigger difference, that such doctors can be identified from existing data that in many cases has already been cleaned but not used for this purpose.(150)

Thirdly, a qualitative study showed that all doctors interviewed knew exceptionally good doctors, that such doctors left a deep impression on them and that exceptionally good doctors may just as likely be vilified as honoured and praised.

Lastly, a survey of the general public showed that most of them knew at least one exceptionally good doctor, one who is exceptional at at least one of diagnosis, treatment or communication, that exceptionally good doctors are statistically substantially different from average doctors (who themselves are already pretty good) except that they are no more popular than average doctors. The one third of exceptionally good doctors that willingly listen to the client to the end stand out even among that group and are considered more knowledgeable and more capable in addition to being better communicators.

Therefore, there are simple, already existing ways to measure the quality of doctors and to improve the quality of doctors such as identifying and learning from exceptionally good doctors. Another obvious example is better management of doctors,(63, 602) a further example is to value them on the level of successful healthcare they provide per dollar spent, which would mean putting general or family practitioners and the research into their work, for example preventative medicine,(91, chapter 12) near the top in terms of prestige when, right now, this part of medicine is at the bottom of the medical hierarchy, and there are many other methods to increase the effectiveness of doctors.

Other research shows in one teaching hospital that hospital doctors that are in the 75th performance percentile of their same-hospital peers (75% of all doctors in the same hospital perform at the same or a lower level than the 75% doctor) save some $2,000 or 5% of costs per hospital admission and have better health results than a 25th performance percentile doctor.(67)

In this context it is seemingly paradoxical that medical students are treated really badly, forcing them to acquire vast amounts of knowledge without looking after them, and then exploiting them as junior doctors, leading to many doctors getting burnt out, quitting or only working part time. This cycle of abuse and exploitation could be ended at any moment but this is not happening.

A reason that makes sense is that that level of demands and exploitation breeds conformism, it is a conditioning for doctors to be too exhausted to have a well-working intuition or to question too many aspects of their environment. A burnt out (depressed at work) doctor is much less likely to challenge the status quo than a vital doctor in full possession of their faculties.

The downside accrues to society at large, losing out on productive members and to the doctors who have elevated levels of suicide(603-605) and burnout with many studies on that subject.(178, 179, 182, 194, 195, 197, 198, 606)

Apart from the mistreatment of medical students and doctors, coming from first principles, it is very strange that the best population health measures, preventative medicine and primary care, are the least prestigious and the least valued parts of medicine with its practitioners the least respected. **Why is knowledge more important than population health?**

In regards to patients, there are preventative interventions that have very high benefit to cost ratios(607) and it may also be valuable to incorporate the insights of behavioural medicine,(608, 609), though this technique has been seriously abused during the recent COVID-19 event.(610-612)

Currently medicine rarely requests the patient to behave in a responsible way even though, for example, chronic diseases are largely preventable. Asking *and knowing how to ask* and supporting patients to be more responsible could well decrease the demands on the overstretched medical system and assist in the healing process itself, making medicine more effective and leading to better outcomes for patients and society as a whole.

The doctors' effect on patients' physical health is ignored and it is actually even more blatant than that – in medical research trials where patients are treated by different doctors, the doctors' influence is mathematically eliminated as much as possible through a technique called multi-level modelling aimed at extracting the influence of the intervention (treatment) from the combined influence of each doctor or 'cluster' as it is termed. In many trials where you have multiple hospitals with multiple doctors in each hospital, the influence of doctors and hospitals (for example, one hospital could have much better nursing staff than another) is not considered separately but only as an effect that needs to be eliminated from the calculations as the focus is on the intervention. Further, as a clinical trial expert advised me privately, in multi-centre randomised controlled trials only the centre is recorded and not the doctor him or herself, thereby ignoring any doctors' effect altogether.

This strikes this author as wasteful. Finding out the value of an intervention is important but finding out the value of a hospital or a particular doctor is also valuable.

Possible causes of this state of affairs may be that:

- nobody has found a way to monetise improving the healing influence of doctors
- there is little demand from doctors to learn how to be less exhausted or to have less burnout
- doctors do not want to be associated with the term 'healers' and little published material is available on this question (doctors as healers) and what there is does not get cited a lot.(613, 614)

It would make sense that there would be great demand from hospitals and governments on ways to reduce burnout for doctors as both suffer a substantial loss when doctors stop working or reduce their working hours. Governments and society also suffer substantial losses if there is a wide range in the quality of hospitals and doctors and sufficient steps are not taken to improve the overall quality.(182, 183, 390, 391, 606, 615, 616)

The Health of Doctors

It is also known that bad mental health of medical students has consequences for their ability to be a doctor,(617) but no attempt has been made to address this vital component and its impact on patient health. As a group, many doctors and other medical staff are highly stressed and overworked(176, 177, 179, 618) and do not look adequately after their own health.(619) There is no systematic approach to investigate the consequences of this stress and overwork or to correct the situation.

As the one presenting with the ill in the first place, it is well known that the patient has a strong influence on the outcome of any medical interaction as there are ongoing efforts at making patients more compliant with their healthcare regime, but again, there is no systematic approach to optimise it.

In other words, we concentrate on one aspect of the medical interaction (the treatment) and get results that are flawed while making it more and more expensive to get these flawed results.

Is there a more ineffective way to improve the number and the results of medical interactions? Is this really the best way to improve population health?

Medical research becomes increasingly expensive and with each scandal loses more and more respect and credibility in the eyes of the public while fewer and urgent problems like the obesity epidemic, diabetes or the rise in cancer incidences are adequately effectively dealt with.

More on Patients

The main focus in medical research regarding patients seems to be about improving compliance and it does not work very well: *"Current methods of improving medication adherence for chronic health problems are mostly complex, labor-intensive, and not predictably effective".*(620)

The Australian Longitudinal Study of Women's Health of currently 57,000 women and active since 1996, shows that, as women get older, they get better at eliminating harmful substances, such as alcohol and smoking, from their life and their compliance rates with healthcare directives are high and either staying high or getting better, but they are unable to improve their daily behaviour when it comes to food and moving their body sufficiently(621)

In the previous reference,(620) this paragraph hints at the reasons:

"At a theoretical level, the nature and determinants of noncompliant behavior are complex and not well understood, although there are interesting models.(622) The following generalizations stem from numerous studies of the determinants of adherence.(210, 622, 623) Compliance has little relation to sociodemographic factors such as age, sex, race, intelligence, and education. Also, although low adherence is a problem with self-administered treatments for all disorders, patients with psychiatric problems are less likely to comply and those with physical disabilities caused by the disease are more likely to comply. In addition, patients tend to miss appointments and drop out of care when there are long waiting times at clinics or long time lapses between appointments. Finally, adherence decreases as the complexity, cost, and duration of the regimen increase."

Educating patients can lead to *"increased involvement in the interaction with the physician, fewer limitations imposed by the disease on patients' functional ability, and increased preference for active involvement in medical decision-making".*(624)

Compliance is a major issue with chronic pain patients.(211) It is not clear what does and does not improve patient compliance. (625) In this meta-analysis *"communication in medical care is highly correlated with better patient adherence".*(626)

The Doctor or Practitioner Again

Compared to the evidence collected on procedures and thera-pies, very little is sought on whether and how doctors make a difference to the healing and treatment process. Hence, doctors are vulnerable to administrators and healthcare payers trying to control how and when they use what intervention through evidence-based medicine.

As there is insufficient evidence on what value doctors add and how they add that value to the equation, there is no check on the impact of new rules and regulations on the work of doc-tors and thus it is not known whether they make doctors less efficient and capable or make them more liable for burnout or terminating their career.

Doctors are also vulnerable to alternative practitioners claiming the latter do a better job as, again, there is not suf-ficient evidence when and how doctors make a difference. This is especially true when a doctor recommends lifestyle changes to a patient that the patient may not be wholly in agreement with.

The Value of Primary Care

An exception to this lack of data is the value of primary care (family doctors or general practitioners) as it is known that comprehensive and family-oriented primary care services sep-arate countries with good health from those with poor health. Also, *"the stronger the primary care, the lower the cost"*.(627)

In other words, the magic weapon to improve healthcare and the cost of healthcare already exists in most countries: Primary care.

Why are these measures not universally adopted? Clearly, there are historical and cultural reasons why healthcare systems have developed the way they have but a very important one is the low status of primary care doctors:

> *"The greatest distinguishing characteristic of primary care medicine—family medicine, general pediatrics, and general internal medicine—is that the subject of care is the person, not a particular disease, not a specific body part, and not just a physical body. Though metaphysics is not a frequent topic of conversation in primary care training programs, all good primary care doctors know that their first responsibility is the ongoing care of the person.*
>
> *This distinction keeps primary care permanently at the bottom of the status hierarchy within academic medical centers.(129) In the arena of modern biomedicine, attempts to integrate the interpersonal aspect of healing into patient care are looked upon, at best, as an extracurricular activity, and not uncommonly with haughty derision—a petty distraction from 'real doctors' concerns with 'real medicine.' This is the legacy of the Flexner Report (628): good medicine defined exclusively in the terms of biomedicine".(91, chapter 12).*

Mistreatment of Trainee Doctors and Established Doctors

When the influence of doctors is misunderstood or ignored,(77) it is only a small step to treating them badly. Working weeks of 80 hours are normal for trainee surgeons. Do we need to cite a reference to show that this is exploitation? However, among senior surgeons the consciousness seems to be that these hours should be increased, as shown in this earlier-mentioned un-ethical study(204) run by very senior surgeons. In other words, surgeons treat each other as what may be described as robots and are behaving as if they were unaware that this may not be desirable and is leading to levels of burnout among 30-38% of surgeons.(180) Burnout in this article is defined as *"emotional exhaustion, depersonalization, and a decreased sense of personal accomplishment"* with younger surgeons being more susceptible to burnout. Burnout can also be described as depression that is limited to working hours.

The results of this surgeons' study(181) are worth quoting in full:

> *"Of the approximately 24,922 surgeons sampled, 7905 (32%) returned surveys. Responders had been in practice 18 years, worked 60 hours per week, and were on call 2 nights/wk (median values), [meaning half have been in practice up to 18 years, the other half 18 years or more, half worked up to 60 hours a week, half worked 60 or more hours a week etc]. Overall, 40% of responding surgeons were burned out, 30% screened positive for symptoms of depression, and 28% had a mental QOL [Quality of Life] score >1/2 standard deviation*

below the population norm [in the bottom 31% of the population]. Factors independently associated with burnout included younger age, having children, area of specialization, number of nights on call per week, hours worked per week, and having compensation determined entirely based on billing [you are more likely to be burnt out if you are younger, have children, are on call more often, work more hours, have no salary and some specialisations are more burnt out than others]. Only 36% of surgeons felt their work schedule left enough time for personal/ family life and only 51% would recommend their children pursue a career as a physician/surgeon."

Here is a group of people who have survived one of the most rigorously selective regimes, work in one of the most prestigious and highly paid professions that is difficult to qualify for if you do not have an interest in people and a strong motivation to be of service to them and yet, only one third felt they had a life beside surgery and half would not recommend their job to others. Would it be correct to assume that aspects of their working conditions must be dire?

A third of the study group returned the survey. The non-respondents may not have had the time or energy to fill it in. Maybe the survey was not designed well or there may be other reasons, like surgeons who are doing well finding there was no need to answer the survey, though a 32% return rate is considered a good rate. If, among the non-respondents, there were many who did not have the time or energy, their distress and despondency may be even worse than among those who did respond to the survey.

Other trainee doctors (residents) also work 80-hour weeks. This regimen leads to more serious medical errors(629) and car crashes for these residents.(630) The hospital providers save money by having every resident perform the work of two doctors but incur the extra costs resulting from serious medical errors. I have not come across a study comparing the costs of these errors with the money saved in doctors' salaries, however, the residents themselves pay a high price, not just in car crashes alone but in the lack of free time for the period of their residency. Other studies report high levels of relationship issues and burnout among them, i.e. the residents suffer long term damage from their stint as trainees.

It may be worth considering that there is a human and a financial cost both to doctors and to patients due to medical errors and, in addition, that the erratic nature of lawsuits makes budgeting particularly difficult for hospitals as one hospital administrator shared with the author in a private conversation.

The cost of treating junior doctors badly may be immense for their quality of life and their effectiveness (burnout, dropouts) as well as for society at large (dropouts, lower standards of care) but may actually even be, most relevantly, higher than doing the opposite for the hospitals concerned, as having doctors who are in bad shape can lead to medical errors and medical errors can have a large human, not just financial cost and lead to substantial suffering that need not have happened.

There are also no conclusive studies the author is aware of that cover the physical and mental consequences and lost lifetime productivity of these physicians as a result of their residency period and very little research that puts a value on doctors' contributions(66, 67) or even that doctors themselves make a difference.(64, 65)

As there is likely no researched and published evidence, the obvious – treating a group of important and very expensive people very badly for years and the ensuing financial consequences – can be ignored with 'progress' being defined to 'limiting' the work weeks of residents to 80 hours except for surgeons.

Treating residents as described is abuse, with senior doctors among the co-conspirators in perpetrating and perpetuating the abuse. Why are senior doctors allowing themselves to participate in this abusive practice of exploiting junior doctors? What is the benefit to them except a grim and twisted form of satisfaction that new doctors are being treated just as badly as they themselves were treated?

What is the purpose to routinely damage a substantial proportion of a group that is among the most expensively educated people on the planet? Isn't this wastage on a grand scale, costing society millions in lost output for each one whose productivity is impaired in the long term through overworking and disempowering junior doctors?

This study(178) found that distress among surgeons is also strongly associated with major medical errors. Could the converse also be true, that well-adjusted surgeons may have improved surgical outcomes? That they will not just have fewer major medical errors but will get a lot of things right their exhausted and burnt-out colleagues may not even notice and that those differences do not show up in the relatively crude statistics that are being collected?

In a "*landmark article*"(631) a surgeon writes about surgical outcomes where certain procedures are used seven or more times as often in some areas of the United States than in others.(632) The more procedures are done, the higher the costs – if you desensitise a group of people (resident surgeons) for a long time, could you end up with some who are not very sensitive to the financial needs of society and have no compunction to overuse procedures that line their pockets, a phenomenon that occurred society-wide in the 1960s to 1980s?(63)

When researching why there is such a regional variance in the number of surgical procedures,(376) the authors found that there is a large grey area where both options, to do the surgery or not, are reasonable decisions,(ibid., pg.1123) leaving the decision to the opinions of the people involved. Could it be possible that a proportion of surgeons might be tempted to make their own earnings one factor affecting those decisions?

In this study(175) about burnout among medical doctors in general we have high rates of distress among doctors, with 46% reporting at least one symptom of burnout. In society in general, people with degrees have lower levels of burnout compared with high school graduates and the higher the degree, the lower the burnout rate. Medical doctors are an exception here as they have a degree as well as substantially higher levels of burnout.

In that same study, the doctors who were in contact with patients the most had the highest levels of burnout, including family and general internal medicine, with two thirds of emergency physicians also suffering burnout. In other words, doctors who deal with a lot or with very distressed patients are particularly in trouble. Clearly, patients can have a strong negative impact on doctors and working with them is making the treating doctors more distressed.

There is also evidence that doctors make more clinical errors with difficult patients,(633) and doctors who are better communicators have a lower patient turnover.(634)

Notwithstanding the above, there does not seem sufficient support for doctors so they can learn how to deal with patients without getting distressed. Some doctors manage, others do not, but those who know how to work with patients without burning out seem unable to sufficiently pass their patient skills on to their colleagues.

There are self-help books for doctors(635) but they do not seem to have a major impact on doctors' behaviour.

As stated earlier, doctors have higher rates of suicide and high rates of burnout. Burnt out and exhausted doctors are less likely to question corruption, unnecessary rules, or intrusive administrators and regulators, reducing the demand for change. Such a system is profoundly inhuman but has developed from the demand or negligence of the various stakeholders.

The British Medical Journal (BMJ) Asked: What Makes a Good Doctor?

The British Medical Journal devoted an entire issue in 2002 to the question "What's a good doctor and how do you make one?". (636) In one article, letters from individual doctors and others who tried to answer this question were published. One illuminating quote among them was:

> *"There is not a single piece of evidence or the means to measure whether a doctor is good or bad".(637)*

Essentially, the letter writers mostly communicated that doctors needed to like people and be good people themselves.

There was not a single mention of a doctor being a role model for their patients.

The editorial of that 2002 issue(601) is very telling: *"… defining a good doctor, I suggest, lies in degree of difficulty somewhere between defining a good composer and a good human being. In fact, it's impossible."* The editorial then comes to the obvious conclusion:

> *"If we cannot define a good doctor, then it is unsurprising that we don't know how to make one. There seems to be some agreement, however, that we are doing poorly at the moment. Medical education may be removing rather than instilling the human qualities that make for a good doctor. We should, say our readers, select the right people and then 'stop them from going rotten through overload, cynicism, and neglect during their training and early career'".*

No suggestion was made how to 'stop them from going rotten'.

Twenty-three years later it seems little has changed with only a handful of research papers(64-67) directly addressing the effect doctors have on patients' physical health as mentioned earlier. Why has nobody else done this research apart from poorly constructed or underpowered surveys?

An oft-cited systematic review found that "physicians who adopt a warm, friendly and reassuring manner are more effective than those who keep consultations formal and do not offer reassurance".(638)

Apart from my research, according to medical research, we do not know what a good doctor is, though 'good doctors' seem to exist, but we cannot distinguish between these good doctors and other doctors; therefore, we do not know how to make good doctors and at the moment it looks as though we are making doctors in their formative stages worse.

The Placebo Effect

The fact is, we have indirectly measured the impact a doctor has on patient health and medical outcomes in at least one way for a long time:

If we assume that good doctors provide better outcomes for the patient than bad doctors, then a doctor is part of the treatment effect. However, if the doctor's part of the treatment effect is considered not to be known, then it must be part of the placebo effect.

The placebo effect is the effect that is left after all known effects have been accounted for.

When we do not know the effect of a doctor, the effect of the doctor must be a part of the unknown. If we assume that the effect is not zero, then the effect of a doctor is part of the unknown, hence the placebo effect.

In other words, one way the quality of a doctor can be measured is by their placebo effect. Doctors whose patients do unusually well presumably are better doctors.

The word 'placebo' comes from the Latin "placebo", which, according to the Oxford English Dictionary (OED)(482), means "*I shall be pleasing or acceptable*". The OED defines the placebo as "*a substance or procedure which a patient accepts as a medicine or therapy but which actually has no specific therapeutic activity for his condition or is prescribed in the belief that it has no such activity*" and the placebo effect as "*a beneficial (or adverse) effect produced by a placebo that cannot be attributed to the nature of the placebo*".

It is difficult to fit the doctor's effect into this definition as his or her work clearly has a therapeutic activity. The Merriam-Webster dictionary's definition is more helpful: The placebo effect is the "*improvement in the condition of a patient that occurs in response to treatment but cannot be considered due to the specific treatment used*".

A 1999 journal article giving a historical overview of placebo and placebo effects,(639) considers the definition of placebo effect more thoroughly and offers four separate definitions, preferring the following one: "*a change in a patient's illness attributable to the symbolic import of a treatment rather than a specific pharmacologic or physiologic property*".(640) This means that no actual material placebo is required. For example, going to the doctor alone can provide a healing.

The Treatment Effect of Doctors

A study(641) of a Norwegian hospital shows that local leadership is important for doctors, nurses and the quality of healthcare as shown by patient outcomes and financial indicators. That 'local leadership' is either from doctors or strongly influenced by doctors.

This vignette from a review of hospital management(642) is worth quoting in full:

> "In the early 1980s the American Nurses' Association identified a group of hospitals that were known by reputation as 'good places to work'. Designated as 'magnet' hospitals because they had little difficulty in recruiting and retaining staff, they were found to share a number of organisational features, including:
>
> + a relatively flat nursing hierarchy with few supervisors;
>
> + the chief nurse had a strong position in the management structure of the hospital;
>
> + nurses had autonomy to make clinical decisions in their own areas of competence and had control over their own practice;

+ decision making was decentralised at the level of the unit;

+ staffing was adequate and limits were placed on the number of new nursing graduates;

+ methods to facilitate communication between nurses and physicians were established;

+ the organisation of nurses' work promoted accountability and continuity of care—for example, primary nursing care;

+ the institution demonstrated the value it attached to nurses—for example, by investing in their education.

Aiken and colleagues at the University of Pennsylvania have since shown in a series of studies that cardinal features of the "magnet" hospitals are related to lower mortality rates, increased patient satisfaction and lower burnout rate and needle stick injuries among nursing staff."

What has this got to do with the quality of doctors? Consider how many of these factors the collective of doctors of those hospitals has an influence on. In addition, senior administrators are often qualified doctors. At least in Australia, hospital management is a recognised specialisation for doctors. A good doctor may not just take care of patients but may also improve all aspects of a hospital with consequent outcomes for everyone there – patients, doctors as well as nursing, auxiliary and administrative staff.

There are studies that show that doctors who, in a children's hospital, make their patients' parents feel met, who are warm and who explain themselves, have patients with better compliance.(643)

The doctor-patient relationship is important in patient compliance(210, 644, 645) and an important variable in other compliance, including the process of prescribing, but it is extremely difficult to assess the nature of this interaction and to measure its components.(646)

There is surprisingly little research on the treatment effects of doctors. It is considered a truism that healthy doctors have healthy patients, but the author could not find research supporting this assertion. There are studies about the effect of doctors' weight on patients(647, 648) and on the effects of healthy habits by the doctors themselves(599, 649, 650) and that being an excellent role model can be taught(651) and that burnout among doctors leads them to reduce their working hours(182) but no studies that measure the treatment effect of doctors and how that can be improved.

One way I studied doctors' performance is not by interviewing patients but by actual treatment results in cohort studies and randomised controlled studies. It turned out that cohort studies could be analysed but large and therefore multi-centre randomised controlled trials do not record the treating doctor, only the centre, making it impossible to analyse doctors' performance. I was surprised at this neglect, but it makes financial sense as clinical trials need more participants for the same statistical power (certainty of result) if doctors have a treatment (clustering) effect themselves.

Cohort studies are very common in education and a meta-analysis of 65,000 research papers comes to the conclusion that 50% of the education outcome is due to the student, 20-25% due to the teacher and the rest of the outcome is distributed quite evenly (6-8% each) among the students' home, their peers, the schools and the principal.(652) Therefore, in education, 70-75% of the variation in outcomes is due to the student and the teacher.

Clearly, medicine is different but the influence of the patient on the healing process is plainly very large as, for example, most chronic diseases are preventable.(653, 654)

The question then becomes why the influence of the doctor is ignored to the degree it is?

It feels very strange that the minutest aspects of interventions are being investigated but it is not even generally known what the influence is of a component that is present in almost all intervention, a human health professional, a component whose influence, depending on the intervention and outcome measured can range from negligible to very large – over 30% of the total variation in patient outcomes, when, for example, aspirin is only responsible for 2% of the total variation in the patient outcome of heart attack(64, 65)

Repeating another example, that component (medical doctor) that is present in very many interventions, in the form of a Norwegian GP can add or subtract, depending on the abilities of the GP, nine months in life expectancy from patients in the first two years of their acquaintance in the case of patients age 55 or older.(66)

Management of Doctors

Many doctors have been enthusiastic proponents of evidence-based medicine even though it gives pharmaceutical and other companies, the health administration bureaucracy and legislators far more power over them than ever before. In return, evidence-based medicine provides a host of useful interventions and makes it easier to get funding for healthcare, as there is evidence that particular investments provide a better health outcome.

However, the disadvantage is that this control by external forces can be and often is misused for the benefit of the external forces and to the detriment of the medical professionals and the patients. Examples are the litigation culture in the United States, which leads to doctors commissioning tests they consider unnecessary, where a false positive (the test says something is wrong but either the test is wrong, as is quite common, or the result is irrelevant as it does not affect the patient's health, or the result detracts from the actual health issue the patient has, causing a delay in treatment) can cause a lot of harm to the patient as such a spurious test result then leads to more tests and possibly interventions (treatments) that damage the patient and were not needed.

Other examples are the health bureaucracy being able to interfere more and more with doctors even before COVID-19 as described in this blog(655) and with the following quotes:

> *"Scientific-bureaucratic medicine seems to be the currently dominant model of EBM in the UK."* and

> *"as the language of EBM becomes ever more*
> *embedded in medical practice, and as bureaucratic*
> *rules become the accepted way to implement 'the*
> *best' evidence, its requirements for evidence are*
> *quietly attenuated in favour of an emphasis on*
> *rules."(656)*

On the other hand, the corruption of over-servicing and over-treating and thereby over-charging in the late 20th century and the demand for over-treatment by patients had to be dealt with as the costs were and are simply unsustainable. As there was substantial resistance to cost control and requests for efficiency, there had to be a counter force reducing costs. (63) That counter force to contain costs is only partially successful as there are also other powerful beneficiaries from over-treating and over-servicing such as pharmaceutical companies which is shown in the steady expansion of the definitions of mental illness(657, 658) and the remuneration of those involved in that expansion.(207)

Medical schools can get away with treating doctors badly and producing burnt out doctors without any direct repercussions and their reputation may not even be affected as medical students rarely are able to compare two or more medical schools.

Hospitals and administrators are able to utterly exploit doctors as the negative consequences of bad treatment on doctors are not measured. Universities can teach medicine with little or no regard to the well-being of the medical students. Patients can dump all their emotions on doctors and demand to be treated without taking any responsibility themselves because there are no substantial initiatives to deal with the harm this attitude does to the patient-facing doctors over time. This harm shows up in the levels of burnout of doctors and doctors resigning from treating patients altogether.

There is research that shows that patients with a very negative attitude receive worse diagnostic care from doctors,(633) but this research could not measure any impact on the doctors' well-being exerted by such patients.

30 Day Mortality Rate by Day of Week

Odds ratio for each day of the week
compared to Monday's 30 day mortality rate

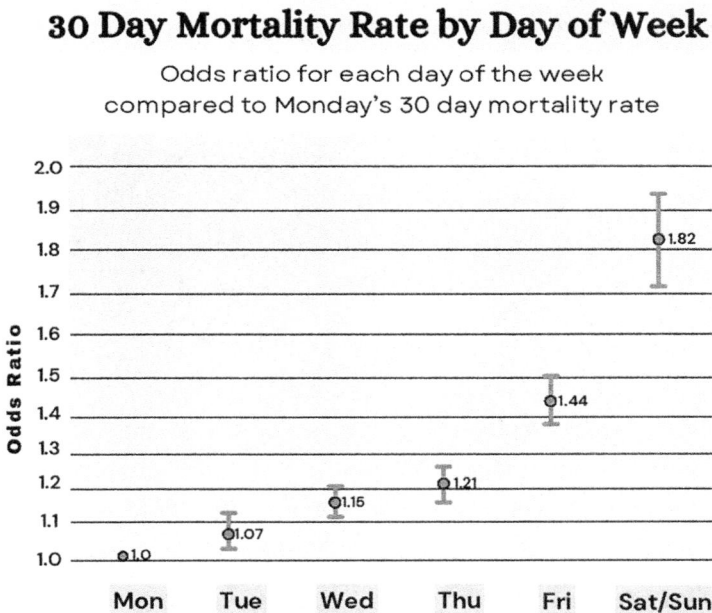

Clearly there are better and worse doctors but, as it turns out(659) individual doctors' performance can change quite dramatically as well, as shown by this graph from the publication displaying the mortality rate due to elective surgery in the UK from 2008-9 to 2010-11 on a weekday basis.

"Adjusted odds of death and 95% confidence intervals by day of procedure in English hospitals for 2008-9 to 2010-11."

'Adjusted odds ratio' means that the researchers made sure that like was compared with like. If for example, poorer people were treated more on Fridays, then the adjustments take care of that effect. Link to video can be found here.(660)

The above chart shows there is a 44% higher chance of dying when the operation is on a Friday (odds ratio of 1.44), than on a Monday. The even higher rate of weekend deaths could be due to other causes as elective surgery normally is not done on a weekend – the weekend volume of elective surgeries is about a quarter of the volume on a weekday. If the elective surgery death rates would have been kept at Monday's level, 4,645 lives would have been saved over the three years of the study. The confidence interval (the vertical line that goes through each dot and ending in two short horizontal lines) shows that the odds ratio for Friday may not be exactly 1.44 but is likely to be between 1.39 and 1.50. For the exact definition you may wish to research "definition of 95% confidence interval" on the internet.

The death rate of elective surgery is 6.7 per 1,000 procedures and the additional mortality for Tuesday to Friday operations is 'only' an extra 1.2 deaths per 1,000 procedures, but the research raises the possibility that other complications may also increase during the week. The important point seems to be that elective surgery teams are getting progressively more tired or exhausted or less attentive for other reasons as the week progresses, hence the current policy of having young doctors work very long hours may have lots of negative consequences not just for doctors but also for patients and possibly the health system as surgical complications are expensive.

In other words, policies that make an effort to reduce or elim-inate tiredness and exhaustion among hospital staff or even doctors outside hospitals may pay for themselves financially as well and quite possibly may be very beneficial financially if fewer doctors leave the profession. There are nurses(661) who have learnt how to deal with and be well despite of and in the midst of workplace stress and have outlined their experience with the stress encountered in hospitals in a submission to Australia's federal parliament.

Bad Doctors

It is better known what makes a bad doctor, with one notorious example being the former GP Harold Shipman, who was Britain's worst serial killer with more than 200 murders. Apart from such an extreme case, it is well-known that doctors at times make bad decisions, some of which have bad consequences and some doctors make more bad decisions than others.

However, according to a 1997 British Medical Journal editori-al(662) *"All doctors are problem doctors"* quoting a book *Problem doctors: a conspiracy of silence,*(663)

> *"[N]o country has an adequate system for managing problem doctors" and "We are all problem doctors. And even if we aren't problem doctors today we might be tomorrow. Who wants to criticise a colleague in such circumstances? We understand how they grapple with the most awful difficulties with limited means, and we don't want to condemn them. We would rather turn away until we are*

forced–by criminal proceedings, publicity, or ghastly consequences for a patient – to act. Then we will, but reluctantly"

and

"Once they arrive, medical students are put through a gruelling course and exposed younger than most of their non-medical friends to death, pain, sickness, and what the great doctor William Osler called the perplexity of the soul. And all this within an environment where 'real doctors' get on with the job and only the weak weep or feel distressed. After qualification, doctors work absurdly hard, are encouraged to tackle horrible problems with inadequate support, and then face a lifetime of pretending that they have more powers than they actually do. And all this within an environment where narcotics and the means to kill yourself are readily available. No wonder some doctors develop serious problems".

This means that in practice, often only the worst offenders are disciplined and everybody else is left to their own devices. This lack of feedback means there is little support available to doctors outside increasing their medical knowledge that allows them to improve their performance.

Patients Again

Patients' bodies respond to more than just the immediate treatment (intervention) in a hospital. The United States government surveys hospital patients and gives hospitals a rating of one to five stars depending on their feedback. The more stars, the fewer complications and the fewer unplanned readmissions.(664) With some procedures, there is little or no difference in complications such as, for example, surgical cuts re-opening when they should not – surgical wound dehiscence, with others the gap is very large (central line-associated bloodstream infection). Unplanned readmissions are strongly connected with these hospital ratings for many procedures.

In the hospital sensory environment a review of studies found that there is little evidence of the hospital environment making much of a difference, at least from the authors' point of view(665) except for music in some circumstances, though many individual studies find effects, including this one with over 3,000 citations.(666)

The following study on social support for people with cancer shows and also lists a number of other studies that people who are isolated where they live or have few people to turn to have lower survival rates when they get cancer. Being married tends to be helpful for survivors with the exception of breast cancer where married women actually fare worse. Being in a support group also helps.(667)

Informed patients make better use of doctors and may assist in their own healing.(624) It is possible to improve patients' adherence to treatments through incentives and reminders but there is no theoretical understanding as to which kind of interventions make some patients adhere better than others.(625)

The patients themselves actually have a big influence on how they perceive their own health. This was shown starkly with colostomy patients who, while they have a colostomy, feel it would be better not to have one but they can live with it. For those who could recover from this condition, they then realised having a colostomy was horrible.(460) Could it be that, because people adjust to their chronic illnesses, the impact of these illnesses may be worse or even much worse than the patients realise, who, in order to cope, minimise their perceived pain and discomfort?

Another reason why patients may minimise their perception of pain and discomfort is so they do not have to take the necessary actions, like changing their lifestyle, what they eat and drink, how much they eat and drink, how much they physically move during the day, how much they need to address any psychological burdens in their life as, as a group, they do not change their behaviour on diagnosis of a chronic disease.(87)

Similarly, patients may minimise their perceived pain and discomfort in order not to be a burden on their environment, either for compassionate reasons or for the environment not to provide feedback to the patients that a change in lifestyle or behaviour may be needed.

A pointer to the possibility that patients are capable of substantially influencing their perception of their overall quality of life is this study(668) where the researchers found that patients' perceived overall quality of life is only weakly correlated (only a little similar) with their doctors' view of the patients' overall quality of life. This lack of a strong relationship between a patient's and their doctor's perception could also be due to the fact that patients are considering their finances and their interpersonal relationships as similarly important for their overall quality of life while the doctor may be less aware of these factors.

Doctors, as they are clinicians, professionally know what to do about burnout and exhaustion, yet a large proportion of doctors are stressed, exhausted and burnt out and, as they know the remedy in great detail, many are choosing to remain stressed, exhausted and burnt out. Would it be surprising if they then are unable to support their patients in being less stressed, exhausted or burnt out?

The Treatment Triangle – The Intervention

In the treatment triangle of the patient, the doctor and the intervention (treatment), each component's influence is important and may be equally important.

Medical research concentrates on the intervention, ignores the doctors and tries to separate the influence of the treatment from the patient's influence on the healing process. If the doctors are very good at improving the health of the patients of a randomised controlled trial (the gold standard in medical research), they will improve the health of both the treatment and control group and this improvement for all participants will be ignored or deemed to be part of the placebo effect. The only item of concern for much of medical research is the difference between the results for the treatment group and the results for the control group. These results are influenced, consciously or unconsciously, by the intent of the researchers, regardless of how much they follow the ever-tightening medical research standards.

It makes business sense to focus on the intervention, as a successful intervention like a new pharmaceutical can be worth a substantial amount of money. The incentives to improve patient responses to treatments or the incentives to reduce a need for the treatment in the first place rest with the entity paying for the healthcare.

This paying entity will either be the patient directly or indirectly by receiving part of their wages as health insurance payments, or the paying entity is the government which is financed by the people.

Governments, for example in Australia, treat preventive medicine or to reduce the need for patients to use healthcare officially as a national priority(621) and they are succeeding with alcohol, smoking and health screening programs like pap smears but not with changes to day-to-day behaviour such as food intake and exercise or daily physical activity. Therefore, the rates of obesity and its consequences like diabetes are increasing. Apart from exhortations by pharmacists for patients to take their pills (who have a financial interest in their exhortation so this may be discounted by the patient), there does not seem to be a substantial number of (or any?) population-wide government initiatives to improve people's adherence to any treatment regimes prescribed by medical doctors.

In other words, there is much less effort spent on the patients' part of the treatment triangle. We have the pharmaceutical

industry and others with strong incentives to financially benefit from interventions against the patient and the government
with opposite incentives to not overpay, that neither patients
nor government perceive as being as strong as the pharmaceutical companies perceive their incentives.

If the pharmaceutical industry's primary concern is about money
and this seems to be the case for at least a subset of the industry
and may well be the dominant concern of the whole industry,(60,
91, 128, 669-672) then the pharmaceutical industry has little incentive for the patient to actually be cured and a strong incentive to
find medication that manages but does not cure chronic disease.

Other indications that money is a dominant influence on the
pharmaceutical industry is the current cost for treatments that
actually provide a valuable cure, like Hepatitis C treatments that
cost some $70,000 in countries that are ready to bear this cost
per treatment(395, 396) but much less in countries that cannot
pay such sums like India where the cost is $900.(673) The pri-
mary motivation seems to be that the pricing in each country is
such as to maximise the revenue for the pharmaceutical company, not the number of patients that can be healed. For example, $900 is currently three months of the average wage in India
which means that a very large number of the estimated 10 million Indian sufferers (0.9% of the 2004 population(674)) miss out.

Dealing With Doctors' Burnout and Stress

There is a lot of research underway to use behavioural science
to 'nudge' people in the right direction but so far no progress
is visible in the chronic disease statistics.

There is no sign of a large-scale discussion on how to reduce burnout and stress among medical professionals. In fact, when research is published that shows that burnout has consequences for healthcare(197) such research can end up being analysed with a fine toothcomb by those with the opinion that burnout does not affect doctors' performance and then forced to be retracted on spurious grounds.(606, 675-677)

Those who become medical professionals must have some impulse to serve and support people as it would be difficult to sustain the arduous training and early clinical years without such an impulse, but the current situation seems to be that this impulse is used, if not exploited, to have doctors and other medical professionals work hard and possibly too hard or to permanently stress them by more work than they can reasonably handle.

The obvious method to reduce the stress levels of doctors and other medical professionals is to reduce their hours or to give them more time with each patient but neither of these are currently realistic as there seems to be a fear such a measure may dramatically raise the cost of healthcare.

One question is why there is so little research or knowledge on how to decrease the stress levels of medical professionals? Some doctors and nurses seem to manage much better than others while working the same hours. How come we do not learn from them in a systematic and widely applicable way?

How come there are only the mildest exhortations or the mildest initiatives for medical professionals to come to work rested, for them to have access to healthy food and to support their management of stress levels and burnout? Are we unaware or are we ignoring that partying hard, as one example, and then working with a hangover, can impede performance?

There is a substantial body of knowledge outside medicine on how to manage people, so they become more productive and enjoy their work more. Why are there so few initiatives to use this knowledge for the help and support of medical professionals? What stops us from making changes that improve productivity by reducing burnout and dropouts among medical professionals and that simultaneously improve their quality of life?

Are medical professionals caught between their impulse to help people and the impossibility to fulfil all the healthcare requests and demands coming from patients, who themselves as a group are behaving irresponsibly? Is the 'solution' adopted by medical professionals to continually display the limits of their ability to deliver, by being genuinely distressed, both physically and mentally?

In other words, are doctors deliberately pushing themselves to and beyond their limits to escape censure from patients who would otherwise say "you are not working hard enough, you could do more for me?" Would this continuous push make doctors then indifferent to the health and well-being of junior doctors, possibly even hostile?

How do overworked and over-stressed doctors react to their exceptionally good colleagues? Some may accept exceptionally good doctors as role models to emulate but, as that is what is happening, many overworked doctors may react with fury and jealousy towards their exceptionally good brethren, allowing regulators and administrators to attack such doctors more easily.(68, 192)

Is the current inadequate care and support for medical professionals a response to them preferring to be in various stages of burnout and exhaustion, as otherwise they would feel even worse, as in, if they were well-rested and enjoying their work immensely, they would be seen by society and their patients as selfish in their impulse to help and support people?

Is it possibly easier to bear being exhausted than being at the receiving end of the jealousy, anger and envy a successful well-adjusted doctor or nurse or other professional in the medical field might attract?

Whether that is true or not, it makes eminent financial sense to take care and preserve or increase the productivity of a highly trained, expensive group of people in society.

If it is possible to improve a medical practitioner's stress level, then such a lifestyle would allow them to be rested and open when the patient enters their practice.

If the practitioner is taking good care, physically and psychologically, of him or herself, they are an obvious role model and they can share their lived wellness with the patient and perhaps even their colleagues. With some practice and experience, these sharings can have a strong impression on patients who are willing to listen. Even patients who are not open are affected when they come across a clear role model, especially a role model who does not impose as it has been shown that role models have an influence on those following them.(678)

There is some scientific understanding about the value of role models for patients, but this does not seem to have been systematically investigated in regard to medical practitioners. There is research on clinicians as role models in teaching medicine(651, 679-682) but not on the impression an obviously healthy doctor who is enjoying their work makes on their patients.

There is much research on the doctor-patient relationship(683) and on patient compliance,(646) but the possibility that a doctor or medical practitioner may have an effect purely based on how they themselves live their life, how much they take care of themselves, how much they enjoy their work, that possibility does not seem to have been considered as a research subject, except for negative medical practitioner role models.

Being lectured on diet (or any medical advice) by an overweight physician(648) or on a healthy lifestyle by a physician whom the patient observed to be smoking at another time or on stress by an obviously tired or rushed physician may not have much of an effect on the patient.

The treatment is clearly important in this triangle and medical science has done a lot of work in amassing a body of knowledge of treatments that work, despite the level of contamination by vested interests and the inherent uncertainty of the process.

The inability of the medical system to successfully teach patients self-care is starting to matter as the number of overweight and obese people is constantly increasing(21, 684) leading in turn to an increase in expensive and debilitating chronic diseases like diabetes.

At present there does not seem to be a recipe to support a population to improve their self-care in two daily matters: What people eat and how much they physically move each day. In fact, following government food recommendations does not seem to have any effect on physical weight in the years that follow(685) and people with higher BMI move less, worsening the problem.(686)

CHAPTER 17

ON THE VASTNESS OF WHAT WE DO NOT KNOW – WHY WE NEED RESEARCH

In its practical application the scientific method has many limitations which are addressed by the scientific community by tightening standards, seemingly with little regard to the cost of these measures.

The Renaissance and the Victorian age had almost non-existent research standards but made great discoveries as they in many ways had few preconceptions about how to find things out, i.e. to do research.

If we still have major gaps in our knowledge as I point out in this chapter, then the tightening of standards, making blue sky research more difficult, could actually be highly detrimental to our scientific understanding of the world. There is also a possibility that some currently unavailable knowledge may have been known at some stage in the past, even though our ability to do research was much less than it is now.

There are many obvious pointers to the major gaps in our knowledge.

Mathematical Pointers to Major Gaps in Our Knowledge

Mathematics made great strides in the 19th and 20th century and many people felt that there was a possibility that eventually "all truths could be proved by self-evident steps from self-evident truths and observation".(687) As it turned out, there are truths that can never be proven but *that are true*. This was first explained by a 25-year-old Austrian, Kurt Gödel in 1931.

Gödel's paradox, or more precisely Gödel's first incompleteness theorem, states:

> "Any consistent formal system F within which a certain amount of elementary arithmetic can be carried out is incomplete"; i.e., there are statements of the language of F which can neither be proved nor disproved in F.(687)

Any scientific research done is carried out within such a formal system F, hence *there are truths that cannot be proven within current research*. In other words, there are three kinds of truths:

- Truths that can be proven via a theorem. An example is Pythagoras's theorem.

- Statements that are accepted as truth because the statistical evidence is sufficient. An example is the statement that smoking causes lung cancer.
- Statements that are true.

The set containing (the collection of) all truths of the first kind is the most constrained, hence this set is smallest in number. The second set is larger but also constrained. The third set is even less constrained so can be expected to be larger, conceivably much larger than the first two sets.

A possible analogy is numbers. The collection of natural numbers "1, 2, 3, ..." is a constrained collection of numbers, even though there is an infinite number of them. The constraint is that they are a fraction where the denominator always has to be 1: "$\frac{1}{1}, \frac{2}{1}, \frac{3}{1}, \frac{4}{1}$...". If the denominator can be any natural number, you end up with an infinite number of fractions for each natural number, for example for the number 2: "$\frac{2}{1}, \frac{2}{2}, \frac{2}{3}, \frac{2}{4}, \frac{2}{5}$,...".

For each fraction, there is an infinite number of transcendent numbers. Examples of famous transcendent numbers are i or π.

Each fraction can be expressed as a recurring decimal number, for example: $\frac{1}{3}$ as $0.\overline{3}$ or 0.33333... or $\frac{3}{2}$ as $1.5\overline{0}$ or 1.500000... or $\frac{1}{7}$ as $0.\overline{142857}$ or 0.142857 142857 142857... The recurrent pattern can be very long and complicated but the pattern has a limited length. If you take a number like 0.142857 that starts with that recurrent pattern but then add an infinite sequence of numbers afterwards that do not recur, you again end up with an infinite amount of numbers for each fraction.

In other words, the fewer constraints you put on a number, the more numbers are there, in fact there are drastically (infinitely) more numbers available for each previous number, each time you remove a constraint.

It may be similar for what is true.

If we only accept something as true when it can be proven by a theorem, we accept only a small fraction of all truths.

If we only accept something that can either be proven by a theorem or to our satisfaction through statistical means, then we have the current state of science that still puts a heavy constraint on what truths are acceptable or not.

It is a bit like saying we will only do mathematics using whole numbers or fractions. We will not allow the usage of transcendental numbers like because they cannot be expressed as fractions. Described that way, the logic makes no sense, yet we accept that same logic in research: We will only accept that which can be proven via a theorem or statistically as truth, in fact in medical research there are attempts to even stop many investigations within this paradigm, such as advocated by the organisation Friends of Science in Medicine.(562)

Until we have a mechanism that reliably allows us to discern what is true and what is not, it makes sense, as an initial, interim step, to only accept truths that can be proven via a theorem or to our satisfaction through statistics.

However, if we do this without the awareness that we are perforce most likely ignoring the vast majority of all truths, then we have a major problem. **We end up with the current situation where we say, "everything that has not been proven will be treated as if it is untrue" and we are not even *looking* for ways to access most truths, in fact we are *rejecting* most truths out of hand.**

That is what is happening in science right now. We are working from the consciousness that, if it cannot be proven statistically, it is worthless. As most published research findings are and have to be false for the many reasons outlined elsewhere in this thesis,(142) we engage in a desperate bid to try to make sure that more and more published research findings are statistically valid because for us only statistically valid research results can be true. We completely ignore that a statistically faulty result could well be true, and we uneasily live with the fact that many statistically valid research results will turn out or have turned out not to be true.

We have accepted statistical validity as a substitute for truth, in fact, apart from theorems, as the only acceptable expression of truth.

The paradoxical and strange result is that when you talk to statisticians about truth, they get very uncomfortable and keep retreating to the concept of statistical validity and do not wish to engage in a discussion whether a scientific finding is true or not.

This is far from a good state of affairs because those who engage statisticians may not be aware that the statistician responds to the question "is there a statistically valid connection here?", while the actual question is "is it true that ...?"

This state of affairs would be less of a problem if both sides are aware of and accept each other's position. It becomes dangerous when a group of people turns this reasoning around and says, "if it cannot be statistically proven, then it will have to be treated as if it is untrue" and try to forbid all medical practices that have not been statistically "proven".

In this approach a lot of clearly false results are labelled as pseudoscience or quackery and rejected, which is desirable, but this approach also rejects what seems to be the vast majority of truths that are not (yet) accessible to the scientific method.

In other words, in evidence-based medicine we are moving towards exclusive acceptance of a tool, scientific research, where most published findings are false and falsified, as the only acceptable tool to practise medicine from. Experience, intuition, heuristics (useful mental shortcuts), expert consensus, anecdotal evidence aka case study and the art of healing do not count, even though experience, intuition, heuristics, expert consensus, anecdotal evidence and the art of healing could well be ways of accessing truths that have not yet been proven statistically. Plainly, experience etc. are often faulty but so is scientific research and there is no evidence that *overall*, either is better and it would seem sensible that a combination of both approaches could be a superior approach.

It is very limiting to declare that there is only one way to access truth when that one way can only ever discern what looks like a small fraction of all truths, where that one way is riddled with errors, in fact where it is the norm that that one way is wrong and where the practitioners themselves, the statisticians, do not want to get involved with truth in the first place but simultaneously enjoy their place as the holders of the rule-book of what can be considered a valid or an invalid result, even though that rulebook leads to faulty results when used in practice and is very easily and thoroughly corrupted.

If we wanted to hide most truths from ourselves without realising we are doing so, we could not have come up with a better system.

In fact, the current system of evidence-based medicine, which is what we are talking about, seems indistinguishable from a system designed to withhold most truths from us. We get interesting and very helpful results from evidence-based medicine, but we could well be missing out on most of what is true.

Evidence pointing into that direction is the obesity epidemic, the increasing levels of exhaustion and mental illness, the aged-adjusted rate of cancer increasing, with other cancers replacing the reduced rate of lung cancer and the fact that life expectancy seems to be plateauing in developed nations and even dropping, as is the case in the UK and in the United States.

Another pointer is that, using the same tools, guidelines and interventions, some doctors are much better in patients' physical health outcomes than their colleagues. Would it be logical to assume that they employ truths in their practice that other doctors do not employ as those truths are not in guidelines or published scientific papers?(64, 65, 68, 192, 688)

A grim way of putting it is that medicine ignores population health by over-emphasising interventions (treatments) and medical research and statistics ignore truth.

Historical evidence of major gaps in our knowledge

A big pointer to knowledge that was available in the past but is not available today is that with our current technology we cannot come close to replicating the pyramids of Giza. There is still no crane that can place stones as heavy as those used in the pyramids with the precision they have been placed in the pyramids.

The pyramids are there. They exist. Therefore, the science that created them existed and could exist again. Science's current attempts to explain the pyramids are to ignore them or to come up with speculative answers. Two examples of attempts are firstly to find a plausible explanation how people with a much lower technology base were able to build them and secondly to come up with an explanation about a much higher-level civilisation in the past, for example through extra-terrestrials.

If the work was done by aliens, there is clearly enormous knowledge that we are missing. If the work was done by humans, there is equally and just as clearly enormous knowledge that we are missing on how to build such monuments without a large technological base.(689).

Areas of Unknown Knowledge

Modern science has very little understanding of death.(690-692)

There are many scientists and medical doctors who smoke and who are obese and these are only the public vices. In addition, a large proportion of doctors suffer from burnout(175-183, 194,

195, 197-200, 390, 391, 606, 615, 616, 618) and suicide rates are higher than for the general population.(603-605)

Evidently there are big gaps between knowledge and the application of that knowledge in our own life. If we do not know how to apply scientific findings in our own life, then we must have extensive gaps in our understanding of ourselves.

If many of us make persistent major errors in how we live our life despite having the knowledge that these activities are harmful to us, then there must be important areas of knowledge that we do not or only incompletely understand.

As even highly sophisticated people engage in self-harming behaviour and that includes those with a thorough understanding of the mind, could there be an important, even decisive influence on us that we are not aware of? There are many theories about this gap between our knowledge and our behaviour but none of these theories gives us an effective way to close that gap.

Why is the age-adjusted rate of cancer increasing? With an ageing population this means that the incidence of cancer is overwhelming our healthcare systems.(494) Why is the prevalence of chronic diseases increasing without abatement, also overwhelming our healthcare system?

For the purposes of this book, the point of scientific knowledge is to get to the truth. That sounds obvious but then why are so many of our actions in scientific research not supportive of getting to the truth?

If knowledge is true knowledge, that is currently considered synonymous with the postulation that the knowledge has been discovered by the scientific method, through evidence-based science. However, there are many reasons as outlined to consider this a very limited approach. There is also knowledge, like the knowledge that built the pyramids, that exists but is currently inaccessible to us.

Is there vastly more scientific knowledge to be found at some stage in the future?

Are there vastly more truths to be found at some stage in the future?

What Is The Point Of Large Undiscovered Areas?

If you examine something that is considered to be largely known, like the geography of a city, it makes sense to spend most of your effort to make sure that the knowledge is accurate. If you examine something that is largely unknown, like North America for the first explorers, it makes sense to increase your knowledge as much as possible and to accept any imperfections in your knowledge which can be fixed over time.

In other words, either approach is the best, depending on the context.

Medical research by its constant tightening of research standards is behaving as if its subject is largely known even though even a cursory examination as shown above makes it clear that there are large, painful and obvious gaps in our knowledge.

This does not mean that we deliberately lower our standards, but we know and accept the unreliability of our research and are open for the truth to present itself in unexpected ways and from unexpected sources beyond the already examined ones such as traditional medicine or indigenous or herbal or Chinese medicine.

Conclusion

Evidence-based medicine is a tool. A very useful tool that has major limitations and has been easily and thoroughly corrupted.

The main weakness is that if you follow the rules then your results are considered to be true. This weakness has led to widespread abuse of the process of scientific research that underpins evidence-based medicine, and the ongoing reaction of tightening research standards is leading to poorer and more expensive research results and increased incentives to be deceptive as research failures have become more expensive.

These weaknesses have their root in the fact that medical research was originally defined as being about diagnoses and treatments and not about the healing, care and well-being of people.

Bringing the focus back on the primacy of population health and accepting that evidence-based medicine is simultaneously the best currently accepted tool to get to truths we have and being aware that evidence-based medicine is nevertheless providing mostly false results, results which cannot be improved beyond a certain point, it makes sense to take stock of what is the best that can be made from a very bad situation.

This acceptance of the actual facts of evidence-based medicine could lead to a far more harmonious usage and implementation of evidence-based medicine, putting the most successful part of healthcare – primary care or family medicine – at the centre.

This point where further tightening of research standards will be more harmful than beneficial may have already been reached. If we accept the intrinsic limitations of research results instead of trying to improve research standards beyond the point of cost effectiveness, then this can lead to a humility that will be far more beneficial to population health than the current situation where research results are mostly accepted at face value and population health is worsening and medical costs are rising at an unsustainable rate.

Therefore, the harm can be limited coming from some of evidence-based medicine's limitations that are intrinsic such as poor quality research findings, guidelines of at times questionable quality and that are often corrupted, evidence-based medicine's inability to deal with multi-symptomatic patients,(120) and its root weakness of replacing a quest for truth with a quest to fulfil rules.

And there is more.

There are two major areas where there is tremendous scope to make healthcare more effective through evidence-based medicine:

1. Further investigating what makes a good doctor and investigating what role and influence the doctor has on the healing process and identifying and learning from exceptionally good doctors. Making doctors more effective and less stressed would be a tremendous boon for the doctors themselves, and society.

2. The people who as a group put in the largest effort to serve humanity, medical doctors, should have a lot more authority than they currently have. They are not cogs that can be replaced at will.

3. How to improve the lifestyle of everyone in society and how to improve patients' adherence to medical treatments. In many cases we have knowledge of what the patient needs to do to stay healthy and to get healthy. What we do not have is how to get patients and people in general to adopt those beneficial practices. Once we find ways for large numbers of people to adopt healthy practices, without abusing that process, as that happened on a grand scale during COVID-19,(56, 245, 246, 610) we can expect a profound improvement in the cost of healthcare and in the quality of life experienced by society.

By making evidence-based medicine much more about people and truth we can tremendously improve the value of evidence-based medicine.

CHAPTER 18

SO WHAT CAN BE DONE ABOUT THE CATASTROPHE THAT IS EVIDENCE-BASED MEDICINE?

There are multiple ways to deal with the discussed design and implementation flaws and corruption of evidence-based medicine with each one leading to improvements of its own. Here are a few examples:

- Currently corrupt or faulty guidelines can cause harm to many people and entire populations at once. Re-empower doctors to be able to override guidelines. Removing the burden of proof on doctors may initially lead to some wrong decisions but will also reduce the impact of false guidelines and create an incentive for guidelines to be of a standard that are voluntarily employed by doctors.

- Require doctors to identify, learn from and not attack but vigorously defend their best peers in order to raise standards.
- Evaluate the cost to society of a doctor quitting or reducing their working hours in the first five years after graduation and incentivise and penalise medical schools and hospitals who abuse junior doctors accordingly. Schools and hospitals that treat their charges badly should experience financial consequences.
- Improve management of healthcare to contain costs as is common in other industries.
- Intensely research under which circumstances patients alter their behaviour towards better health and routinely require and support a measure of lifestyle responsibility.
- Reduce the reporting and other requirements for clinical trials so that clinical trials can be run more often and more cheaply, allowing more blue-sky research and therefore increasing the number of unexpected positive medical trial outcomes.
- Encourage evidence-based medicine to have as its aim improved population health in addition to individual health outcomes. This could have the immediate effect of substantially or even massively upgrading the appreciation and valuation of primary care which is GPs, family physicians, nurses and other trained professionals as that seems the cheapest and most effective way to improve an entire population's health.

We can learn to live with uncertainty and that research on interventions (treatments) is deeply biased, therefore we should not focus on the tightening of research standards to the detriment of beneficial health outcomes. The focus needs to be on improved medical interactions and outcomes.

Ultimately, medical research is about improving the health of people, it is not about anything else. Focusing on one aspect of improving the health of people inevitably means that other aspects get ignored or ill attended to. If these other aspects have any importance in the health of people, then we are diminishing their health compared to where it could be and possibly diminishing it on an absolute basis.

For example, by allowing patients to behave much more irresponsibly than is advisable for them when it comes to diet,{Who, #199}(621, 693-696) patients are left alone to such a degree that not even chronic diseases alter their behaviour on a population basis with those who improve their behaviour being offset by those worsening their behaviour.(87)

Most importantly, learn how to ask and support the patient to behave responsibly, as the pressure from patients' irresponsible demands is the root of much of the difficulties we have with healthcare.

We can acknowledge that we are getting less and less value from evidence-based medicine and medical spending in general and that research results are inherently of low quality and that it is difficult or impossible to improve the quality in a cost-effective way.

In this(567) article from the New England Journal of Medicine the authors show that the cost to increase the life expectancy of a person by a year through medical care has gone up by a factor of 6 for a newborn to a factor of 12 for a 65 year old in inflation adjusted dollars from 1960 to 2000.

It cost, adjusted for inflation, $14,000 in 2002 dollars to increase the life of a newborn by a year through medical care in 1960 and $83,000 in 2000. For 65-year-olds the figures are $11,500 and $147,000.

Currently the accepted answer to medical issues is more research that is of seemingly better quality. Simply acknowledging that more and better research is only a small part of the answer for increased population health can steer resources into more effective approaches as outlined in this chapter.

Only change the rules of how to do the research part of evidence-based medicine if on balance they lead to more knowledge and understanding of the world, i.e. useful research findings, do not just look at what needs to be stopped, look at the costs of stopping it and look for measures that have benefits in outcomes and reduce the costs of research.

STOP ignoring that the whole process of evidence-based medicine is easily corruptible and that this corruption is pervasive and either take the corruption into account while it is still pervasive or take steps to reduce the corruption or the incentives to be corrupt. This includes accountability.

It is entirely possible to work within a corrupt system as an individual while keeping one's integrity, doing what needs doing and using what freedom and truthful information is available.

An example during COVID-19 is referring to research that shows that higher Vitamin D levels are associated with lower suscepti- bility to respiratory diseases, that zinc plus a zinc ionophore, i.e. a compound that is not antiviral in itself but allows zinc, which is an antiviral when it enters cells, to enter cells in an infected body, that zinc plus an ionophore such as the over-the-coun- ter Quercetin has had good research results, that intravenous Vitamin C is associated with faster recovery,(40) that the risk of COVID-19 is negligible for children and youths and small for healthy people(39, 697, 698) and that there were no mRNA in- jections used as vaccines prior to COVID-19 that were consid- ered to be non-controversially safe.(699-701)

There is also substantial scope for improving the value for money received in the research of interventions as that pro- cess has so far been run will little regard to costs and benefits. This is a well-accepted truism as shown in a special 2014 issue of Lancet,(440, 442, 470, 471, 473) though the remedies proposed here – mostly more rules – will not deliver less wastage. Mi- chael Millenson(63) gives good examples on how to make the implementation of healthcare more efficient.

We need to include doctors as being equally important to interventions in medical research.

Consider whether the current, almost exclusive emphasis on in- terventions while mostly ignoring the influence of the doctor and the patient on the healing process, is sufficient or whether inves- tigating the doctor and patient as follows could be worthwhile:

Find out in much greater detail what makes good doctors and who they are.(64-67, 150) Support and learn from those that have superior patient outcomes. That can raise standards in ways that the large majority of doctors can appreciate and enjoy. It is more fun when we can do a good job.

Additionally, make it easier for doctors to take care of their physical and mental health. This need not mean fewer working hours, except for junior doctors in hospitals. It can be as simple as providing healthy food in the canteen, making sugar less available, offering doctors ways to work while using fewer stimulants such as caffeine and sugar by offering them programs to stop being exhausted and cease demanding that they follow rules that they know are harmful and demoralise them.

There are of course many other issues in this area to include such as the constant threats of litigation and the influence of drug companies and those with vested interests. All of the above have an eroding effect on the doctors and medical staff.

Hence, medical doctors need a much stronger and more assertive lobby to defend their patients' rights and their own rights to enable better patient care. Yes, it is likely that self-interest can and will take over but the experience of being wholly subsumed to other, often corrupt forces in the last 40 years may have a cautionary effect on self-serving demands and it is less likely that the grand corruption of the current system will be continued on the same scale when those who actually treat patients have more say. It is quite shocking that the doctors' abdication of their duty to represent patients and themselves have allowed other vested interest such as the media, government, legislators and pharmaceutical companies to take over as completely as they have.

Study the long-term productivity effects and costs to society of exploiting junior doctors in hospitals and incentivise medical schools and hospitals to do better once the financial consequences of the abuse are known. If there is a control group of young doctors who have not been subjected to such long hours (or to fewer long hours), use a longitudinal study, whether prospective (going forward) or retrospective (looking at existing data), to ascertain the impact on their future productivity through factors such as burnout or leaving healthcare altogether. There may well be enough existing data to do a retrospective study, and expressing the difference between the two groups in dollars lost to society per doctor may make the decision makers in healthcare review their position if the difference is large.

If that is difficult, simply surveying doctors on their off-duty behaviour during their internship years and then ascertaining which factors have a detrimental effect on doctors' physical and mental health. Possible options are binge drinking or "partying hard", doing further studies while exhausted, being unable to deal with traumatic situations, having sleep issues etc.

Even if only doctors are available for research who are going through the crucible of overly long clinical hours, it is possible to check their physical and mental health and to follow their careers to see if there are levels of exhaustion or other distress that exponentially affect their future effectiveness as doctors by forcing them to reduce or eliminate their practising hours down the track. A simple way of putting it may be to see if junior doctors as a group recover from burnout and exhaustion as they get older or if the symptoms worsen.

In many ways, it is conceptually simple. Consider doctors a long-term asset and use well-known strategies to preserve, maintain and support these assets. In other words, treat them like humans, with good care and they may respond with being able to provide good care for themselves and their patients.

Find role models of other healthcare workers that are highly effective. Find out which of the skills of these role models are transferable and, if yes, measure the effect on productivity.

Simply use modern management methods with a particular eye for the long term.

Most doctors start out with a love for people and a strong impulse to serve people. This commitment is needed as the study and training is long and arduous. There can be other reasons to become a doctor such as the good income, family pressures or to find out about an ailment they themselves or a person close to them has. Research how prevalent a desire to be of service to humanity is among new students and if, how and why they change over the years. Such research can have a big influence simply by providing feedback to management and teaching staff of the consequences of their actions.

Taking measures that remove the triggers that harden the students' and young doctors' attitudes may be helpful. This does not mean making the medical training easier but, for example, making strategies to study part of the curriculum easier to learn. Perform economic research calculating the short-, medium- and long-term costs to the doctors and to society of doctors dropping out, changing professions, being burnt out and committing suicide. Once something is measured, it can be managed. Currently it is not known how expensive bad quality medical training and exploitative hospital working arrangements are for the persons concerned and for society.

Above all, make population health, people, truth and well-being, not interventions, the purpose of evidence-based medicine.

ABOUT THE AUTHOR

Christoph Schnelle, PhD is a medical researcher and epidemiologist.

Christoph has extensive experience in research, business, finance and applied software development. He is the first author of 10 medical research papers and five patents with some 500 citations as of 2024. He has a Masters in Medical Statistics and a PhD in Health Science and Medicine.

In addition to the above Christoph has nine financial planning qualifications and owns and runs both an Australia wide Financial Planning business and an Australian Financial Services Licensee – this gives him many insights into what motivates people and through the insurance side of the business hears much about people's medical condition and life style. In addition he has many medical professionals as clients and friends.

Christoph is famous for his BBQ lamb becoming a great cook later in life. He lives and works in Australia, inland from Byron Bay with Nicola, his beautiful wife and partner in all things.

References

1. Sackett DL, Rosenberg WMC, Gray JAM, Haynes RB, Richardson WS. Evidence based medicine: what it is and what it isn't. BMJ. 1996;312(7023):71. Available from: http://www.bmj.com/content/312/7023/71.abstract.

2. Stubbs T, Kentikelenis A, Gabor D, Ghosh J, McKee M. The return of austerity imperils global health. BMJ Global Health. 2023;8(2):e011620. Available from: https://gh.bmj.com/content/bmjgh/8/2/e011620.full.pdf.

3. ÓhAiseadha C, Quinn GA, Connolly R, Wilson A, Connolly M, Soon W, et al. Unintended Consequences of COVID-19 Non-Pharmaceutical Interventions (NPIs) for Population Health and Health Inequalities. International Journal of Environmental Research and Public Health. 2023;20(7):5223. Available from: https://www.mdpi.com/1660-4601/20/7/5223.

4. Venkataramani AS, O'Brien R, Tsai AC. Declining Life Expectancy in the United States: The Need for Social Policy as Health Policy. JAMA. 2021;325(7):621-2. Available from: https://doi.org/10.1001/jama.2020.26339.

5. Sampson L, Kubzansky LD, Koenen KC. The Missing Piece: A Population Health Perspective to Address the U.S. Mental Health Crisis. Daedalus. 2023;152(4):24-44. Available from: https://doi.org/10.1162/daed_a_02030.

6. Montez JK. US State Polarization, Policymaking Power, and Population Health. Milbank Q. 2020;98(4):1033-52. Available from: https://pmc.ncbi.nlm.nih.gov/articles/PMC7772643/.

7. Zang E, Lynch SM, West J. Regional differences in the impact of diabetes on population health in the USA. J Epidemiol Community Health. 2021;75(1):56-61. Available from: https://pmc.ncbi.nlm.nih.gov/articles/PMC8128513/.

8. Walsh D, Dundas R, McCartney G, Gibson M, Seaman R. Bearing the burden of austerity: how do changing mortality rates in the UK compare between men and women? Journal of Epidemiology and Community Health. 2022;76(12):1027-33. Available from: https://jech.bmj.com/content/jech/76/12/1027.full.pdf.

9. Jakovljevic M, Timofeyev Y, Ranabhat CL, Fernandes PO, Teixeira JP, Rancic N, et al. Real GDP growth rates and healthcare spending – comparison

between the G7 and the EM7 countries. Globalization and Health. 2020;16(1):64. Available from: https://doi.org/10.1186/s12992-020-00590-3.

10. Matthew McGough AW, Shameek Rakshit, Krutika Amin,. Health System Tracker [Internet]: healthsystemtracker.org. 2023. [cited 2024]. Available from: https://www.healthsystemtracker.org/chart-collection/u-s-spending-healthcare-changed-time/#Total%20national%20health%20 expenditures,%20US%20$%20Billions,%201970-2022.

11. Laviana AA, Luckenbaugh AN, Resnick MJ. Trends in the Cost of Cancer Care: Beyond Drugs. J Clin Oncol. 2020;38(4):316-22. Available from: https:// www.ncbi.nlm.nih.gov/pmc/articles/PMC6994251/.

12. Micah Hartman ABM, Joseph Benson, Aaron Catlin,. National Health Care Spending In 2018: Growth Driven By Accelerations In Medicare And Private Insurance Spending. Health Affairs. 2020;39(1):8-17. Available from: https://www.healthaffairs.org/doi/abs/10.1377/hlthaff.2019.01451.

13. Dieleman JL, Cao J, Chapin A, Chen C, Li Z, Liu A, et al. US Health Care Spending by Payer and Health Condition, 1996-2016. JAMA. 2020;323(9):863-84. Available from: https://doi.org/10.1001/jama.2020.0734.

14. Nunn R, Parsons J, Shambaugh J. A dozen facts about the economics of the US health-care system. The Hamilton Project, Economic Facts. 2020. Available from: https://www.brookings.edu/wp-content/uploads/2020/03/ HealthCare_Facts_WEB_FINAL.pdf.

15. Mikić Z. [Imhotep--builder, physician, god]. Med Pregl. 2008;61(9-10):533-8. Available from: http://europepmc.org/abstract/MED/19203075.

16. IQVIA Institute for Human Data Science. Global Trends in R&D 2023. 2023 February 2023. Available from: https://www.iqvia.com/insights/the-iqvia-institute/ reports-and-publications/reports/global-trends-in-r-and-d-2023.

17. Masic I, Miokovic M, Muhamedagic B. Evidence based medicine - new approaches and challenges. Acta Inform Med. 2008;16(4):219-25. Available from: https://pmc.ncbi.nlm.nih.gov/articles/PMC3789163/.

18. Angelakis AN, Vuorinen HS, Nikolaidis C, Juuti PS, Katko TS, Juuti RP, et al. Water Quality and Life Expectancy: Parallel Courses in Time. Water. 2021;13(6):752. Available from: https://www.mdpi.com/2073-4441/13/6/752.

19. Hertz E, Hebert JR, Landon J. Social and environmental factors and life expectancy, infant mortality, and maternal mortality rates: Results of a cross-national comparison. Soc Sci Med. 1994;39(1):105-14. Available from: https://www.sciencedirect.com/science/article/abs/pii/0277953694901708.

20. Howick J. Exploring the asymmetrical relationship between the power of finance bias and evidence. Perspect Biol Med. 2019;62(1):159-87. Available from: https://www.scopus.com/inward/record.uri?eid=2-s2.0-85065432820&doi=10.1353%2fpbm.2019.0009&partnerID=40&md5=5479 3df75bb4e012298676c00525784a.

21. Gomersall S, Dobson A, Brown W. Weight gain, overweight, and obesity: determinants and health outcomes from the Australian Longitudinal Study

on Women's Health. Current obesity reports. 2014;3(1):46-53. Available from: https://www.ncbi.nlm.nih.gov/pubmed/26626467.

22. Schopenhauer A. Die Welt als Wille und Vorstellung (German, in Foreword): Penguin Random House Verlagsgruppe FSC® N001967; 1859. 93 p. Available from: http://www.zeno.org/Philosophie/M/Schopenhauer,+Arthur/Die +Welt+als+Wille+und+Vorstellung/Erster+Band/%5BVorreden%5D.

23. Kennedy Jr RF. The real Anthony Fauci: Bill Gates, Big Pharma, and the Global War on Democracy and Public Health: Simon and Schuster; 2023.

24. Kennedy Jr RF. The Wuhan Cover-Up

    And the Terrifying Bioweapons Arms Race. New York: Skyhorse Publishing, Children's Health Defense; 2023.

25. Chang G. NIH Funded China's Gain-of-Function Research at the Wuhan Institute of Virology. August; 2021. Available from: https://centerforsecuritypolicy.org/ wp-content/uploads/2021/08/Chang_NIH-1.pdf.

26. Jonathan Calvert, George Arbuthnott. What really went on inside the Wuhan lab weeks before Covid erupted. Sunday Times. 2023. Available from: https://tritorch.com/degradation/Whatreallywentoninside theWuhanlabweeksbeforeCoviderupted.pdf.

27. Alistair Dawber. Covid escaped from Wuhan lab, US report finds. The Times. 2023. Available from: https://tritorch.com/degradation/ WhatreallywentoninsidetheWuhanlabweeksbeforeCoviderupted.pdf.

28. Looi M-K. Did covid-19 come from a lab leak in China? BMJ. 2023;382:p1556. Available from: https://www.bmj.com/content/bmj/382/bmj.p1556.full. pdf.

29. Burki T. Ban on gain-of-function studies ends. The Lancet Infectious Diseases. 2018;18(2):148-9. Available from: https://www.thelancet.com/ journals/laninf/article/PIIS1473-30091830006-9/fulltext.

30. David E. Martin. The Fauci/COVID-19 Dossier2021. Available from: https:// www.covidtruths.co.uk/wp-content/uploads/2021/04/The-FauciCOVID-19-Dossier2532.pdf.

31. Bruttel V, Washburne A, VanDongen A. Endonuclease fingerprint indicates a synthetic origin of SARS-CoV-2. bioRxiv. 2023:2022.10.18.512756. Available from: https://www.biorxiv.org/content/biorxiv/early/ 2023/04/11/2022.10.18.512756.full.pdf.

32. Segreto R, Deigin Y, McCairn K, Sousa A, Sirotkin D, Sirotkin K, et al. Should we discount the laboratory origin of COVID-19? Environmental Chemistry Letters. 2021;19(4):2743-57. Available from: https://doi.org/10.1007/ s10311-021-01211-0.

33. National Institutes of Health. Statement on Funding Pause on Certain Types of Gain-of-Function Research [August 7]. 2014 [updated 2024. Available from: https://www.nih.gov/about-nih/who-we-are/nih-director/statements/ statement-funding-pause-certain-types-gain-function-research.

34. BBC News Reality Check team. Coronavirus: Was US money used to fund risky research in China?2021 2024. Available from: https://www.bbc.com/news/57932699.

35. Eban K, Vanity Fair. In Major Shift, NIH Admits Funding Risky Virus Research in Wuhan2021 2024. Available from: https://www.vanityfair.com/news/2021/10/nih-admits-funding-risky-virus-research-in-wuhan.

36. Miller AM, Fox News. NIH acknowledges US funded gain-of-function at Wuhan lab, despite Fauci's denials2021 2024. Available from: https://www.foxnews.com/politics/nih-acknowledges-us-funded-gain-of-function-wuhan-lab-despite-faucis-denials.

37. Sharon Lerner, Mara Hvistendahl. New Details Emerge About Coronavirus Research at Chinese Lab2021 2024. Available from: https://theintercept.com/2021/09/06/new-details-emerge-about-coronavirus-research-at-chinese-lab/

     https://archive.md/aayAN.

38. Sharon Lerner, First Look Institute. The Intercept v. National Institutes of Health2021 2024. Available from: https://archive.md/BUAGt#selection-407.0-407.46.

39. Ioannidis JPA. Infection fatality rate of COVID-19 inferred from seroprevalence data. Bull World Health Organ. 2021;99(1):19-33f. Available from: https://pubmed.ncbi.nlm.nih.gov/33716331/.

40. C19 Collective. COVID-19 early treatment: real-time analysis of 4,357 studies 2024 [Available from: https://c19early.org/.

41. Mathieu E, Ritchie H, Ortiz-Ospina E, Roser M, Hasell J, Appel C, et al. A global database of COVID-19 vaccinations. Nature Human Behaviour. 2021;5(7):947-53. Available from: https://doi.org/10.1038/s41562-021-01122-8.

42. Data OWi. COVID-19 vaccine doses administered by manufacturer

     All doses, including boosters, are counted individually.: Our World In Data. org; 2024. Available from: https://ourworldindata.org/grapher/covid-vaccine-doses-by-manufacturer?country=European+Union~URY~USA~ARG~CAN~CHL~ECU~HKG~JPN~NPL~NOR~PER~ZAF~KOR~CHE~UKR.

43. Fraiman J, Erviti J, Jones M, Greenland S, Whelan P, Kaplan RM, et al. Serious adverse events of special interest following mRNA COVID-19 vaccination in randomized trials in adults. Vaccine. 2022;40(40):5798-805. Available from: https://www.sciencedirect.com/science/article/pii/S0264410X22010283.

44. Thorp JA, Thorp MM, Thorp EM, Scott-Emuakpor A, Thorp KE. Global COVID-19 Pandemic Outcomes: A Cross-Country Comparison Study of Policy Strategies. Integrative Medicine: A Clinician's Journal. 2024;23(2):46-53. Available from: https://search.ebscohost.com/login.aspx?direct=true&AuthType=shib&db=ccm&AN=178099039&site=ehost-live&custid=s1097571.

45. Kirsch S, Marik P, Rogers C, Cosgrove K, Mead MN. A Novel Practical Approach for Directly Assessing COVID-19 Vaccine Efficacy against Hospitalization2024. Available from: https://doi.org/10.20944/preprints202408.0338.v1.

46. Bellavite P, Ferraresi A, Isidoro C. Immune Response and Molecular Mechanisms of Cardiovascular Adverse Effects of Spike Proteins from SARS-CoV-2 and mRNA Vaccines. Biomedicines. 2023;11(2):451. Available from: https://www.mdpi.com/2227-9059/11/2/451.

47. Lee Y, Jeong M, Park J, Jung H, Lee H. Immunogenicity of lipid nanoparticles and its impact on the efficacy of mRNA vaccines and therapeutics. Experimental & Molecular Medicine. 2023;55(10):2085-96. Available from: https://doi.org/10.1038/s12276-023-01086-x.

48. Giannotta G, Murrone A, Giannotta N. COVID-19 mRNA Vaccines: The Molecular Basis of Some Adverse Events. Vaccines. 2023;11(4):747. Available from: https://www.mdpi.com/2076-393X/11/4/747.

49. Acevedo-Whitehouse K, Bruno R. Potential health risks of mRNA-based vaccine therapy: A hypothesis. Medical Hypotheses. 2023;171:111015. Available from: https://www.sciencedirect.com/science/article/pii/S0306987723000117.

50. Rubio-Casillas A, Rodriguez-Quintero CM, Redwan EM, Gupta MN, Uversky VN, Raszek M. Do vaccines increase or decrease susceptibility to diseases other than those they protect against? Vaccine. 2024;42(3):426-40. Available from: https://www.sciencedirect.com/science/article/pii/S0264410X23015062.

51. Kuhbandner C, Reitzner M. Differential Increases in Excess Mortality in the German Federal States During the COVID-19 Pandemic. 2024. Available from: https://blog.fdik.org/2024-03/state-comparism-researchgate_p.pdf.

52. Alessandria M, Malatesta GM, Berrino F, Donzelli A. A Critical Analysis of All-Cause Deaths during COVID-19 Vaccination in an Italian Province. Microorganisms. 2024;12(7):1343. Available from: https://www.mdpi.com/2076-2607/12/7/1343.

53. Allen DW. Covid-19 Lockdown Cost/Benefits: A Critical Assessment of the Literature. International Journal of the Economics of Business. 2022;29(1):1-32. Available from: https://doi.org/10.1080/13571516.2021.1976051.

54. Daryarana K. 2020. Available from: https://www.heritage.org/public-health/commentary/failures-influential-covid-19-model-used-justify-lockdowns.

55. Jefferson T, Dooley L, Ferroni E, Al-Ansary LA, van Driel ML, Bawazeer GA, et al. Physical interventions to interrupt or reduce the spread of respiratory viruses. Cochrane Database of Systematic Reviews. 2023(1). Available from: https://doi.org//10.1002/14651858.CD006207.pub6.

56. Sandlund J, Duriseti R, Ladhani SN, Stuart K, Noble J, Høeg TB. Child mask mandates for COVID-19: a systematic review. Archives of disease in childhood. 2024;109(3):e2-e. Available from: https://adc.bmj.com/content/109/3/e2.abstract

https://web.archive.org/web/20231212074504id_/https://adc.bmj.com/content/archdischild/early/2023/12/02/archdischild-2023-326215.full.pdf.

57. Joffe AR. SARS-CoV-2, COVID-19, and Children: Myths and Evidence. In: Beckwith S, editor. Update in Pediatrics. Cham: Springer International Publishing; 2023. p. 503-20. Available from: https://doi.org/10.1007/978-3-031-41542-5_20.

58. Dance A. The shifting sands of 'gain-of-function' research. Nature. 2021;598:554-7. Available from: https://www.nature.com/articles/d41586-021-02903-x.

59. Evans I, Thornton H, Chalmers I, Glasziou P. Testing treatments: better research for better healthcare. 2011.

60. Gøtzsche PC. Deadly medicines and organised crime: how Big Pharma has corrupted healthcare: Radcliffe Publishing Ltd;; 2013.

61. Gøtzsche PC. Our prescription drugs kill us in large numbers. Pol Arch Med Wewn. 2014;124(11):628-34. Available from: https://goldengalaxies.net/Quasar/wp-content/uploads/2022/12/Our-prescription-drugs-kill-us-in-large-numbers-Article-October-30-2014-Peter-C.-Gotzsche.pdf.

62. Gøtzsche P, Winn D. Psychiatry beyond repair

    Conversations. HUMAN GIVENS. 2023;30(2-2023):28. Available from: https://www.scientificfreedom.dk/wp-content/uploads/2023/12/Denise-Win-Human-Givens-Peter-Gotzsche-interview.pdf.

63. Millenson ML. Demanding medical excellence: Doctors and accountability in the information age: University of Chicago Press; 2018.

64. Schnelle C, Clark J, Mascord R, Jones M. Is there a doctors' effect on patients' physical health, beyond the intervention and all known factors? A systematic review. Ther Clin Risk Manag. 2022;18:721-37. Available from: https://www.dovepress.com/is-there-a-doctors-effect-on-patients-physical-health-beyond-the-inter-peer-reviewed-fulltext-article-TCRM.

65. Schnelle C, Clark J, Mascord R, Jones M. Is There a Surgeons' Effect on Patients' Physical Health, Beyond the Intervention, That Requires Further Investigation? A Systematic Review. Ther Clin Risk Manag. 2022(18):467-90. Available from: https://www.dovepress.com/is-there-a-surgeons-effect-on-patients-physical-health-beyond-the-inte-peer-reviewed-fulltext-article-TCRM.

66. Cicala S, Lieber EMJ, Marone V. Does Your Doctor Matter? Doctor Quality and Patient Outcomes2022 2024. Available from: https://www.cesifo.org/en/publications/2022/working-paper/does-your-doctor-matter-doctor-quality-and-patient-outcomes.

67. Fletcher JM, Horwitz LI, Bradley E. Estimating the Value Added of Attending Physicians on Patient Outcomes. National Bureau of Economic Research Working Paper Series. 2014;No. 20534. Available from: http://www.nber.org/papers/w20534.

68. Schnelle C, Jones MA. Qualitative Study of Medical Doctors on Their Experiences and Opinions of the Characteristics of Exceptionally Good Doctors. Adv Med Educ Pract. 2022;13:717-31. Available from: https://doi.org/10.2147/AMEP.S370980.

69. Hedge Z. "Being A Doctor And Courageous Runs In My Family" - The French Scientist Behind Hydroxychloroquine 2024 [updated October 12th, 2023. Available from: https://www.zerohedge.com/markets/being-doctor-and-courageous-runs-my-family-french-scientist-behind-hydroxychloroquine.

70. Willsher K. Covid: controversial French professor Didier Raoult stands firm on hydroxychloroquine [August 7]. 2020 [updated 2024. Available from: https://www.theguardian.com/world/2020/nov/12/covid-professor-didier-raoult-hydroxychloroquine.

71. Gorski D. COVID-19 antivax quacks are now repurposing ivermectin for cancer [August 7]. 2023 [updated 2024. Available from: https://sciencebasedmedicine.org/covid-19-antivax-quacks-are-now-repurposing-ivermectin-for-cancer/.

72. Brueck H. Why ivermectin is being used to treat COVID-19, and the 2 doctors who are leading the charge [August 7]. 2021 [updated 2024. Available from: https://www.businessinsider.com/why-ivermectin-being-used-treat-covid-2-doctors-leading-charge-2021-9.

73. Ainsworth-Vaughn N. Claiming power in doctor-patient talk: Oxford University Press, USA; 1998.

74. Katz J. The silent world of doctor and patient: Jhu Press; 2002.

75. Albury C, Webb H, Ziebland S, Aveyard P, Stokoe E. What happens when patients say "no" to offers of referral for weight loss? - Results and recommendations from a conversation analysis of primary care interactions. Patient Education and Counseling. 2022;105(3):524-33. Available from: https://www.sciencedirect.com/science/article/pii/S0738399121005619.

76. Pilnick A, Dingwall R. On the remarkable persistence of asymmetry in doctor/patient interaction: A critical review. Social Science & Medicine. 2011;72(8):1374-82. Available from: https://www.sciencedirect.com/science/article/pii/S0277953611001213.

77. Djulbegovic B, Schnelle C. RE: EBM 2.0- from averages to individualized decision -making.... EVIDENCE-BASED-HEALTH: JISCMAIL.AC.UK; 2023. Available from: https://www.jiscmail.ac.uk/cgi-bin/wa-jisc.exe?A2=ind2308&L=EVIDENCE-BASED-HEALTH&O=D&P=36312.

78. Woodhill JM, Palmer AJ, Leelarthaepin B, McGilchrist C, Blacket RB. Low Fat, Low Cholesterol Diet in Secondary Prevention of Coronary Heart Disease. In: Kritchevsky D, Paoletti R, Holmes WL, editors. Drugs, Lipid Metabolism, and Atherosclerosis. Boston, MA: Springer US; 1978. p. 317-30. Available from: https://doi.org/10.1007/978-1-4684-0967-3_18.

79. Frantz ID, Dawson EA, Ashman PL, Gatewood LC, Bartsch GE, Kuba K, et al. Test of effect of lipid lowering by diet on cardiovascular risk. The Minnesota Coronary Survey. Arteriosclerosis: An Official Journal of the American Heart Association, Inc. 1989;9(1):129-35. Available from: https://www.ahajournals.org/doi/abs/10.1161/01.ATV.9.1.129.

80. Ramsden CE, Zamora D, Leelarthaepin B, Majchrzak-Hong SF, Faurot KR, Suchindran CM, et al. Use of dietary linoleic acid for secondary prevention of coronary heart disease and death: evaluation of recovered data from the Sydney Diet Heart Study and updated meta-analysis XX. BMJ. 2013;346. Available from: http://www.bmj.com/content/bmj/346/bmj.e8707.full.pdf.

81. Ramsden CE, Zamora D, Majchrzak-Hong S, Faurot KR, Broste SK, Frantz RP, et al. Re-evaluation of the traditional diet-heart hypothesis: analysis

of recovered data from Minnesota Coronary Experiment (1968-73) XX. BMJ. 2016;353. Available from: http://www.bmj.com/content/bmj/353/bmj.i1246.full.pdf.

82. Johnson RJ, Segal MS, Sautin Y, Nakagawa T, Feig DI, Kang D-H, et al. Potential role of sugar (fructose) in the epidemic of hypertension, obesity and the metabolic syndrome, diabetes, kidney disease, and cardiovascular disease2. The American Journal of Clinical Nutrition. 2007;86(4):899-906. Available from: https://www.sciencedirect.com/science/article/pii/S0002916523135052.

83. Hu FB. Resolved: there is sufficient scientific evidence that decreasing sugar-sweetened beverage consumption will reduce the prevalence of obesity and obesity-related diseases. Obesity Reviews. 2013;14(8):606-19. Available from: http://dx.doi.org/10.1111/obr.12040.

84. Luger M, Lafontan M, Bes-Rastrollo M, Winzer E, Yumuk V, Farpour-Lambert N. Sugar-Sweetened Beverages and Weight Gain in Children and Adults: A Systematic Review from 2013 to 2015 and a Comparison with Previous Studies. Obesity Facts. 2017;10(6):674-93. Available from: https://www.karger.com/DOI/10.1159/000484566.

85. Siegel RL, Miller KD, Wagle NS, Jemal A. Cancer statistics, 2023. Ca Cancer J Clin. 2023;73(1):17-48. Available from: https://acsjournals.onlinelibrary.wiley.com/doi/full/10.3322%2Fcaac.21763

   https://www.researchgate.net/profile/Nikita-Sandeep-Wagle/publication/367077576_Cancer_Statistics_2023/links/63c06a9a4804ba12ffbf3a70/Cancer-Statistics-2023.pdf.

86. My Two Cents. The List of Members of the Young Global Leaders & Global Leaders for Tomorrow of the World Economic Forum: 1993-2022 Volume 1 - Ordered by Member Name: My Two Cents,; 2023 23 January 2023. 118 p.

87. Dontje ML, Krijnen WP, de Greef MH, Peeters GG, Stolk RP, van der Schans CP, et al. Effect of diagnosis with a chronic disease on physical activity behavior in middle-aged women. Preventive medicine. 2016;83:56-62. Available from: https://www.sciencedirect.com/science/article/abs/pii/S0091743515003667

   https://pure.rug.nl/ws/portalfiles/portal/12727510/Complete_dissertation.pdf.

88. Diamond DM, Ravnskov U. How statistical deception created the appearance that statins are safe and effective in primary and secondary prevention of cardiovascular disease. Expert review of clinical pharmacology. 2015;8(2):201-10. Available from: https://www.tandfonline.com/doi/abs/10.1586/17512433.2015.1012494

   https://cardiacos.net/wp-content/uploads/ArticulosMedicos/20180920/2015-How-statistical-deception-created-the-appearance-that-statins-are-safe-an-deffective-in-primary-and-secondary-prevention-of-cardiovascular-disease.pdf.

89. Han BH, Sutin D, Williamson JD, Davis BR, Piller LB, Pervin H, et al. Effect of statin treatment vs usual care on primary cardiovascular prevention among older adults: The ALLHAT-LLT randomized clinical trial. JAMA

Internal Medicine. 2017;177(7):955-65. Available from: https://www.scopus.com/inward/record.uri?eid=2-s2.0-85021307572&doi=10.1001%2fjamainternmed.2017.1442&partnerID=40&md5=ba5f404f4c65d8b25c6ffd3527e6a457.

90. Kristensen ML, Christensen PM, Hallas J. The effect of statins on average survival in randomised trials, an analysis of end point postponement. BMJ Open. 2015;5(9). Available from: http://bmjopen.bmj.com/content/5/9/e007118.abstract.

91. Abramson J. Overdosed America: The broken promise of American medicine: Harper Collins; 2008.

92. Danza P KT, Haddix M, et al. . SARS-CoV-2 Infection and Hospitalization Among Adults Aged ≥18 Years, by Vaccination Status, Before and During SARS-CoV-2 B.1.1.529 (Omicron) Variant Predominance — Los Angeles County, California, November 7, 2021–January 8, 2022. CDC; 2022. Available from: https://www.cdc.gov/mmwr/volumes/71/wr/mm7105e1.htm#suggestedcitation.

93. Griffin JB HM, Danza P, et al. SARS-CoV-2 Infections and Hospitalizations Among Persons Aged ≥16 Years, by Vaccination Status — Los Angeles County, California, May 1–July 25, 2021. CDC; 2022. Available from: https://www.cdc.gov/mmwr/volumes/70/wr/mm7034e5.htm.

94. Marion F. Gruber, Ramachandra Naik, CAPT Michael Smith, Susan Wollersheim, Nabil Al-Humadi, Lei Huang, et al. Emergency Use Authorization (EUA) for an Unapproved Product Review Memorandum. Pfizer; 2020. Available from: https://www.fda.gov/media/144416/download.

95. Brownell KD, Warner KE. The Perils of Ignoring History: Big Tobacco Played Dirty and Millions Died. How Similar Is Big Food? Milbank Quarterly. 2009;87(1):259-94. Available from: http://dx.doi.org/10.1111/j.1468-0009.2009.00555.x.

96. Qaseem A, Wilt TJ. Disclosure of Interests and Management of Conflicts of Interest in Clinical Guidelines and Guidance Statements: Methods From the Clinical Guidelines Committee of the American College of Physicians. Annals of Internal Medicine. 2019;171(5):354-61. Available from: https://www.acpjournals.org/doi/abs/10.7326/M18-3279.

97. Choudhry NK, Stelfox H, Detsky AS. Relationships between authors of clinical practice guidelines and the pharmaceutical industry. JAMA. 2002;287(5):612-7. Available from: http://dx.doi.org/10.1001/jama.287.5.612.

98. Grilli R, Magrini N, Penna A, Mura G, Liberati A. Practice guidelines developed by specialty societies: the need for a critical appraisal. The Lancet. 2000;355(9198):103-6. Available from: http://www.sciencedirect.com/science/article/pii/S0140673699021716.

99. Lenzer J. Why we can't trust clinical guidelines. BMJ : British Medical Journal. 2013;346. Available from: https://www.bmj.com/content/bmj/346/bmj.f3830.full.pdf.

100. Leiß O. 2015 – 2020 dietary guidelines for americans – End of the low-fat,low-cholesterol era? Verdauungskrankheiten. 2016;34(5):229-43. Available from: https://www.researchgate.net/profile/Ottmar-Leiss/

publication/309670933_2015_-_2020_dietary_guidelines_for_americans_-_End_of_the_low-fatlow-cholesterol_era/links/59b663daa6fdcc3f88994723/2015-2020-dietary-guidelines-for-americans-End-of-the-low-fat-low-cholesterol-era.pdf.

101. Cosgrove L, Peters SM, Vaswani A, Karter JM. Institutional corruption in psychiatry: Case analyses and solutions for reform. Social and Personality Psychology Compass. 2018;12(6):e12394. Available from: https://compass.onlinelibrary.wiley.com/doi/abs/10.1111/spc3.12394.

102. Rodwin MA. Institutional Corruption and the Pharmaceutical Policy. Journal of Law, Medicine & Ethics. 2013;41(3):544-52. Available from: https://www.cambridge.org/core/product/C0AEA73FC2D33EAEFBB38F64ECDA388B.

103. Lessig L. "Institutional Corruption" Defined. The Journal of Law, Medicine & Ethics. 2013;41(3):553-5. Available from: https://journals.sagepub.com/doi/abs/10.1111/jlme.12063

      https://papers.ssrn.com/sol3/Delivery.cfm?abstractid=2295067.

104. Fields G. Corruption of Pharmaceutical Markets: Addressing the Misalignment of Financial Incentives and Public Health. The Journal of Law, Medicine & Ethics. 2013;41(3):571-80. Available from: https://www.cambridge.org/core/journals/journal-of-law-medicine-and-ethics/article/abs/corruption-of-pharmaceutical-markets-addressing-the-misalignment-of-financial-incentives-and-public-health/B0AC613BC1AEDDC85AA58B9EA2F439B7

      https://papers.ssrn.com/sol3/Delivery.cfm?abstractid=2286415.

105. Jorgensen PD. Pharmaceuticals, Political Money, and Public Policy: A Theoretical and Empirical Agenda. The Journal of Law, Medicine & Ethics. 2013;41(3):561-70. Available from: https://www.cambridge.org/core/journals/journal-of-law-medicine-and-ethics/article/abs/pharmaceuticals-political-money-and-public-policy-a-theoretical-and-empirical-agenda/861CFA025BABCC50776CD6265335A4B8

      https://papers.ssrn.com/sol3/Delivery.cfm?abstractid=2292148.

106. Gagnon M-A. Corruption of Pharmaceutical Markets: Addressing the Misalignment of Financial Incentives and Public Health. The Journal of Law, Medicine & Ethics. 2013;41(3):571-80. Available from: https://www.cambridge.org/core/journals/journal-of-law-medicine-and-ethics/article/abs/corruption-of-pharmaceutical-markets-addressing-the-misalignment-of-financial-incentives-and-public-health/B0AC613BC1AEDDC85AA58B9EA2F439B7

      https://papers.ssrn.com/sol3/Delivery.cfm?abstractid=2286415.

107. Light DW, Lexchin J, Darrow JJ. Institutional Corruption of Pharmaceuticals and the Myth of Safe and Effective Drugs. The Journal of Law, Medicine & Ethics. 2013;41(3):590-600. Available from: https://www.cambridge.org/core/journals/journal-of-law-medicine-and-ethics/article/abs/institutional-corruption-of-pharmaceuticals-and-the-myth-of-safe-and-effective-drugs/12BBDFC13802D1BD4DA3D7473DD7EBDE

      https://papers.ssrn.com/sol3/Delivery.cfm?abstractid=2282014.

108. Brown A. Key Opinion Leaders and the Corruption of Medical Knowledge: What the Sunshine Act Will and Won't Cast Light on. The Journal of Law, Medicine & Ethics. 2013;41(3):635-43. Available from: https://onlinelibrary.wiley.com/doi/abs/10.1111/jlme.12073

https://papers.ssrn.com/sol3/Delivery.cfm?abstractid=2272672.

109. Cosgrove L, Wheeler EE. Drug Firms, the Codification of Diagnostic Categories, and Bias in Clinical Guidelines. The Journal of Law, Medicine & Ethics. 2013;41(3):644-53. Available from: https://www.cambridge.org/core/journals/journal-of-law-medicine-and-ethics/article/abs/drug-firms-the-codification-of-diagnostic-categories-and-bias-in-clinical-guidelines/C2DC02279A6134B0AD4FD11992AB6CE0

https://papers.ssrn.com/sol3/Delivery.cfm?abstractid=2286724.

110. Rodwin MA. Rooting Out Institutional Corruption to Manage Inappropriate Off-Label Drug Use. The Journal of Law, Medicine & Ethics. 2013;41(3):654-64. Available from: https://onlinelibrary.wiley.com/doi/abs/10.1111/jlme.12075

https://papers.ssrn.com/sol3/Delivery.cfm?abstractid=2309079.

111. Rose SL. Patient Advocacy Organizations: Institutional Conflicts of Interest, Trust, and Trustworthiness. The Journal of Law, Medicine & Ethics. 2013;41(3):680-7. Available from: https://www.proquest.com/scholarly-journals/patient-advocacy-organizations-institutional/docview/2730835400/se-2?accountid=14723.

112. Sommersguter-Reichmann M, Wild C, Stepan A, Reichmann G, Fried A. Individual and Institutional Corruption in European and US Healthcare: Overview and Link of Various Corruption Typologies. Applied Health Economics and Health Policy. 2018;16(3):289-302. Available from: https://doi.org/10.1007/s40258-018-0386-6.

113. Ibrahim J, Majoor J. Corruption in the health care system: the circumstantial evidence. Australian Health Review. 2002;25(2):20-6. Available from: https://www.publish.csiro.au/paper/AH020020.

114. García PJ. Corruption in global health: the open secret. The Lancet. 2019;394(10214):2119-24. Available from: https://doi.org/10.1016/S0140-6736(19)32527-9.

115. Krumholz HM, Radford MJ, Wang Y, Chen J, Heiat A, Marciniak TA. National Use and Effectiveness of β-Blockers for the Treatment of Elderly Patients After Acute Myocardial InfarctionNational Cooperative Cardiovascular Project. JAMA. 1998;280(7):623-9. Available from: https://doi.org/10.1001/jama.280.7.623.

116. Mitchell JB, Ballard DJ, Whisnant JP, Ammering CJ, Samsa GP, Matchar DB. What Role Do Neurologists Play in Determining the Costs and Outcomes of Stroke Patients? Stroke. 1996;27(11):1937-43. Available from: https://www.ahajournals.org/doi/abs/10.1161/01.STR.27.11.1937.

117. Bradley J. From 'trust us, we're doctors' to the rise of evidence-based medicine. The Conversation; 2012. Available from: https://findanexpert.

unimelb.edu.au/news/22217-from-'trust-us--we're-doctors'-to-the-rise-of-evidence-based-medicine.

118. Sackett DL. Evidence-based medicine: Wiley Online Library; 2000. Available from: https://onlinelibrary.wiley.com/doi/10.1002/0470011815.b2a08019

https://pubmed.ncbi.nlm.nih.gov/9190027/.

119. Greenhalgh T. How to read a paper: The basics of evidence-based medicine: John Wiley & Sons; 2014.

120. Greenhalgh T, Howick J, Maskrey N. Evidence based medicine: a movement in crisis? BMJ. 2014;348. Available from: http://www.bmj.com/bmj/348/bmj.g3725.full.pdf.

121. Sheridan DJ, Julian DG. Achievements and Limitations of Evidence-Based Medicine. Journal of the American College of Cardiology. 2016;68(2):204-13. Available from: http://www.sciencedirect.com/science/article/pii/S0735109716331370.

122. Greenlee RT, Murray T, Bolden S, Wingo PA. Cancer statistics, 2000. CA: A Cancer Journal for Clinicians. 2000;50(1):7-33. Available from: https://acsjournals.onlinelibrary.wiley.com/doi/abs/10.3322/canjclin.50.1.7.

123. Kearns CE, Schmidt LA, Glantz SA. Sugar industry and coronary heart disease research: A historical analysis of internal industry documents. JAMA Internal Medicine. 2016. Available from: http://dx.doi.org/10.1001/jamainternmed.2016.5394.

124. Malik VS, Popkin BM, Bray GA, Després J-P, Willett WC, Hu FB. Sugar-Sweetened Beverages and Risk of Metabolic Syndrome and Type 2 Diabetes: A meta-analysis. Diabetes Care. 2010;33(11):2477-83. Available from: https://doi.org/10.2337/dc10-1079.

125. Kearns CE, Apollonio D, Glantz SA. Sugar industry sponsorship of germ-free rodent studies linking sucrose to hyperlipidemia and cancer: An historical analysis of internal documents. PLOS Biology. 2017;15(11):e2003460. Available from: https://doi.org/10.1371/journal.pbio.2003460.

126. Moss M. Salt, sugar, fat: how the food giants hooked us: Random House; 2013.

127. Veldheer S, Yingst J, Zhu J, Foulds J. Ten-year weight gain in smokers who quit, smokers who continued smoking and never smokers in the United States, NHANES 2003–2012. International Journal of Obesity. 2015;39(12):1727-32. Available from: https://doi.org/10.1038/ijo.2015.127.

128. Moynihan R, Gøtzsche PC, Heath I, Henry D. Selling sickness: the pharmaceutical industry and disease mongering

Commentary: Medicalisation of risk factors. BMJ. 2002;324(7342):886-91. Available from: https://www.bmj.com/content/bmj/324/7342/886.1.full.pdf.

129. Block SD, Clark-Chiarelli N, Peters AS, Singer JD. Academia's chilly climate for primary care. JAMA. 1996;276(9):677-82. Available from: http://dx.doi.org/10.1001/jama.1996.03540090023006.

130. World Health Organization, Unicef. Primary health care: a joint report. 1978. Available from: https://www.who.int/publications/i/item/9241800011.

131. Macinko J, Starfield B, Shi L. Quantifying the Health Benefits of Primary Care Physician Supply in the United States. International Journal of Health Services. 2007;37(1):111-26. Available from: https://journals.sagepub.com/doi/abs/10.2190/3431-G6T7-37M8-P224.

132. Basu S, Berkowitz SA, Phillips RL, Bitton A, Landon BE, Phillips RS. Association of Primary Care Physician Supply With Population Mortality in the United States, 2005-2015. JAMA Intern Med. 2019;179(4):506-14. Available from: https://pubmed.ncbi.nlm.nih.gov/30776056/

https://www.researchgate.net/publication/331183855_Association_of_Primary_Care_Physician_Supply_With_Population_Mortality_in_the_United_States_2005-2015.

133. Orzylowska EM, Jacobson JD, Bareh GM, Ko EY, Corselli JU, Chan PJ. Food intake diet and sperm characteristics in a blue zone: A Loma Linda Study. European Journal of Obstetrics Gynecology and Reproductive Biology. 2016;203:112-5. Available from: https://www.sciencedirect.com/science/article/abs/pii/S0301211516302615

https://www.carnivoreisvegan.com/wp-content/uploads/2019/07/Food-intake-diet-and-sperm-characteristics-in-a-blue-zone.pdf.

134. Fisher B, Montague E, Redmond C, Barton B, Borland D, Fisher ER, et al. Comparison of radical mastectomy with alternative treatments for primary breast cancer: A first report of results from a prospective randomized clinical trial. Cancer. 1977;39(6):2827-39. Available from: http://dx.doi.org/10.1002/1097-0142(197706)39:6<2827::AID-CNCR2820390671>3.0.CO;2-I

https://tinyurl.com/nhke5ehz.

135. Kuriakose D, Xiao Z. Pathophysiology and Treatment of Stroke: Present Status and Future Perspectives. International Journal of Molecular Sciences. 2020;21(20):7609. Available from: https://www.mdpi.com/1422-0067/21/20/7609.

136. Gideon Lewis-Kraus. They Studied Dishonesty. Was Their Work a Lie? The New Yorker. 2023. Available from: https://www.newyorker.com/magazine/2023/10/09/they-studied-dishonesty-was-their-work-a-lie.

137. Simonsohn U, Nelson L, Simmons J. [112] Data Falsificada (Part 4): "Forgetting The Words" 2024 [Available from: https://datacolada.org/.

138. Simmons J. [118] Harvard's Gino Report Reveals How A Dataset Was Altered 2024 [Available from: https://datacolada.org/.

139. Cohen D. FDA official: "clinical trial system is broken". BMJ : British Medical Journal. 2013;347:f6980. Available from: https://www.bmj.com/content/bmj/347/bmj.f6980.full.pdf.

140. Hooker RC. The rise and rise of evidence-based medicine. The Lancet. 1997;349(9061):1329-30. Available from: http://www.sciencedirect.com/science/article/pii/S0140673605625524.

141. Upshur RE, Tracy CS. Legitimacy, authority, and hierarchy: Critical challenges for evidence-based medicine. Brief Treatment & Crisis Intervention. 2004;4(3). Available from: https://www.researchgate. net/profile/Ross-Upshur/publication/31504222_Legitimacy_Authority_ and_Hierarchy_Critical_Challenges_for_Evidence-Based_Medicine/ links/0046353bd110349015000000/Legitimacy-Authority-and-Hierarchy-Critical-Challenges-for-Evidence-Based-Medicine.pdf.

142. Ioannidis JPA. Why most published research findings are false. PLoS Med. 2005;2(8):0696-701. Available from: https://journals.plos.org/ plosmedicine/article?id=10.1371/journal.pmed.0020124.

143. Cabana MD, Rand CS, Powe NR, et al. Why don't physicians follow clinical practice guidelines?: A framework for improvement. JAMA. 1999;282(15):1458-65. Available from: http://dx.doi.org/10.1001/jama.282.15.1458.

144. Neuman J, Korenstein D, Ross JS, Keyhani S. Prevalence of financial conflicts of interest among panel members producing clinical practice guidelines in Canada and United States: cross sectional study. BMJ. 2011;343:d5621. Available from: https://www.bmj.com/content/bmj/343/bmj.d5621.full. pdf.

145. Carlisle A, Bowers A, Wayant C, Meyer C, Vassar M. Financial Conflicts of Interest Among Authors of Urology Clinical Practice Guidelines. European Urology. 2018;74(3):348-54. Available from: https://www.sciencedirect. com/science/article/pii/S0302283818303294.

146. Tabatabavakili S, Khan R, Scaffidi MA, Gimpaya N, Lightfoot D, Grover SC. Financial Conflicts of Interest in Clinical Practice Guidelines: A Systematic Review. Mayo Clinic Proceedings: Innovations, Quality & Outcomes. 2021;5(2):466-75. Available from: https://www.sciencedirect.com/science/ article/pii/S2542454820302009.

147. Woolf SH, Grol R, Hutchinson A, Eccles M, Grimshaw J. Clinical guidelines: potential benefits, limitations, and harms of clinical guidelines. Bmj. 1999;318(7182):527-30. Available from: https://www.bmj.com/ content/318/7182/527.short.

148. Perlis RH, Perlis CS, Wu Y, Hwang C, Joseph M, Nierenberg AA. Industry sponsorship and financial conflict of interest in the reporting of clinical trials in psychiatry. American Journal of Psychiatry. 2005. Available from: https://psychiatryonline.org/doi/full/10.1176/appi.ajp.162.10.1957

https://psychiatryonline.org/doi/pdf/10.1176/appi.ajp.162.10.1957.

149. Havighurst CC. Practice Guidelines as Legal Standards Governing Physician Liability. Law and Contemporary Problems. 1991;54(2):87-117. Available from: http://www.jstor.org/stable/1191739.

150. Schnelle C, Jones MA. The doctors' effect on patients' physical health outcomes beyond the intervention. A methodological review. Clin Epidemiol. 2022;14:851-70. Available from: https://www.tandfonline.com/doi/ full/10.2147/CLEP.S357927

https://www.tandfonline.com/doi/pdf/10.2147/CLEP.S357927.

151. Branch AaHCS. National Ambulatory Medical Care Survey: 2018 National Summary Tables. In: (NCHS) NCfHS, editor. 2018. Available from: https://www.cdc.gov/nchs/data/ahcd/namcs_summary/2018-namcs-web-tables-508.pdf.

152. Health AGDo. Medicare in Australia 2022 [Available from: https://www.aihw.gov.au/reports/primary-health-care/medicare-subsidised-care-2022-23/contents/gp-attendances

   https://www.aihw.gov.au/reports/primary-health-care/general-practice-allied-health-primary-care.

153. c19 Collective. c19hcq.org HCQ for COVID-19: real-time meta analysis of 421 studies 2024 [Available from: https://c19hcq.org/.

154. c19 Collective. c19ivm.org Remdesivir for COVID-19: real-time meta analysis of 72 studies 2024 [Available from: https://c19early.org/s.

155. C19 Collective. c19ivm.org Molnuparivir for COVID-19: real-time meta analysis of 20 studies 2024 [Available from: https://c19early.org/m.

156. c19 Collective. c19ivm.org Outcomes in COVID-19 paxlovid studies 2024 [Available from: https://c19early.org/plmeta.html.

157. Bailey CL, Birch L, McDowell DG. PCR: Factors Affecting Reliability and Validity: Royal Society of Chemistry: Cambridge, UK; 2008.

158. Velavan TP, Meyer CG. COVID-19: A PCR-defined pandemic. International Journal of Infectious Diseases. 2021;103:278-9. Available from: https://doi.org/10.1016/j.ijid.2020.11.189.

159. Lenzer J, Hoffman JR, Furberg CD, Ioannidis JPA. Ensuring the integrity of clinical practice guidelines: a tool for protecting patients. BMJ : British Medical Journal. 2013;347:f5535. Available from: https://www.bmj.com/content/bmj/347/bmj.f5535.full.pdf.

160. Xie Y, Wang K, Kong Y. Prevalence of Research Misconduct and Questionable Research Practices: A Systematic Review and Meta-Analysis. Science and Engineering Ethics. 2021;27(4):41. Available from: https://doi.org/10.1007/s11948-021-00314-9.

161. Fanelli D. How Many Scientists Fabricate and Falsify Research? A Systematic Review and Meta-Analysis of Survey Data. PLOS ONE. 2009;4(5):e5738. Available from: https://doi.org/10.1371/journal.pone.0005738.

162. Lexchin J, Bero LA, Djulbegovic B, Clark O. Pharmaceutical industry sponsorship and research outcome and quality: systematic review. BMJ. 2003;326(7400):1167-70. Available from: https://www.bmj.com/content/326/7400/1167

   http://www.bmj.com/content/bmj/326/7400/1167.full.pdf.

163. Upshur REG. Looking for rules in a world of exceptions: Reflections on evidence-based practice. Perspect Biol Med. 2005;48(4):477-89. Available from: http://muse.jhu.edu/article/188207.

164. Haynes RB. What kind of evidence is it that Evidence-Based Medicine advocates want health care providers and consumers to pay attention

to? BMC Health Services Research. 2002;2(1):3. Available from: https://doi.org/10.1186/1472-6963-2-3.

165. Horton R. Common sense and figures: the rhetoric of validity in medicine (Bradford Hill Memorial Lecture 1999). Statistics in Medicine. 2000;19(23):3149-64. Available from: https://onlinelibrary.wiley.com/doi/abs/10.1002/1097-0258%2820001215%2919%3A23%3C3149%3A%3AAID-SIM617%3E3.0.CO%3B2-E.

166. Greenhalgh T, Snow R, Ryan S, Rees S, Salisbury H. Six 'biases' against patients and carers in evidence-based medicine. BMC Medicine. 2015;13(1):1-11. Available from: http://dx.doi.org/10.1186/s12916-015-0437-x.

167. Hanin L. Why statistical inference from clinical trials is likely to generate false and irreproducible results. BMC Medical Research Methodology. 2017;17(1):127. Available from: https://doi.org/10.1186/s12874-017-0399-0.

168. Kelly MP, Heath I, Howick J, Greenhalgh T. The importance of values in evidence-based medicine. BMC Medical Ethics. 2015;16(1):69. Available from: https://doi.org/10.1186/s12910-015-0063-3.

169. Michael Allen. News & Perspectives [Internet]: Medscape. 2022. [cited 2024]. Available from: https://www.idse.net/Covid-19/Article/08-21/MDs-Spreading-COVID-Vaccine-Misinformation-Risk-Losing-Medical-Licenses/64365.

170. Therapeutic Goods Administration. New restrictions on prescribing ivermectin for COVID-19. In: Care DoHaA, editor. 2020 and 2021. Available from: https://www.tga.gov.au/news/media-releases/new-restrictions-prescribing-ivermectin-covid-19.

171. Credentialing Resource Centre. News & Analysis [Internet]: Credentialing Resource Centre. 2021. [cited 2024]. Available from: https://credentialing resourcecenter.com/articles/physician-loses-license-over-covid-19-misinformation.

172. Schluger NW, Prager K. A License to Practice Medicine Cannot Be a License to Harm. Am J Med. 2022;135(8):e229-e30. Available from: https://www.amjmed.com/article/S0002-9343(22)00144-9/fulltext.

173. Wampold BE, Imel ZE. The great psychotherapy debate: The evidence for what makes psychotherapy work: Second edition
Chapter 6 Therapist Effect: Taylor and Francis Inc.; 2015. 1-323 p.

174. Baldwin SA, Imel Z. Therapist effects: Findings and methods. Bergin and Garfield's handbook of psychotherapy and behavior change. 2013;6:258-97.

175. Shanafelt TD, Boone S, Tan L, Dyrbye LN, Sotile W, Satele D, et al. Burnout and satisfaction with work-life balance among US physicians relative to the general US population. Archives of internal medicine. 2012;172(18):1377-85. Available from: https://jamanetwork.com/journals/jamainternalmedicine/fullarticle/1351351

176. Arigonia F, Bovierb PA, Sappinoa A-P. Trend in burnout among Swiss doctors. 2010. Available from: https://smw.ch/index.php/smw/article/view/1165

https://smw.ch/index.php/smw/article/download/1165/1214.

177. Prins JT, Hoekstra-Weebers JE, Gazendam-Donofrio SM, Dillingh GS, Bakker AB, Huisman M, et al. Burnout and engagement among resident doctors in the Netherlands: a national study. Medical education. 2010;44(3):236-47. Available from: https://asmepublications.onlinelibrary.wiley.com/doi/abs/10.1111/j.1365-2923.2009.03590.x

https://core.ac.uk/download/pdf/148192284.pdf.

178. Shanafelt TD, Balch CM, Bechamps G, Russell T, Dyrbye L, Satele D, et al. Burnout and Medical Errors Among American Surgeons. Annals of Surgery. 2010;251(6):995-1000. Available from: http://journals.lww.com/annalsofsurgery/Fulltext/2010/06000/Burnout_and_Medical_Errors_Among_American_Surgeons.1.aspx.

179. Soler JK, Yaman H, Esteva M, Dobbs F, Group EGPRNBS. Burnout in European family doctors: the EGPRN study. Family practice. 2008. Available from: https://academic.oup.com/fampra/article-abstract/25/4/245/606286

https://citeseerx.ist.psu.edu/document?repid=rep1&type=pdf&doi=6422968e92bf8a54f8798127f9ec8419b72afa59.

180. Balch CM, Freischlag JA, Shanafelt TD. Stress and burnout among surgeons: understanding and managing the syndrome and avoiding the adverse consequences. Archives of surgery. 2009;144(4):371-6. Available from: https://jamanetwork.com/journals/jamasurgery/fullarticle/404847.

181. Shanafelt TD, Balch CM, Bechamps GJ, Russell T, Dyrbye L, Satele D, et al. Burnout and Career Satisfaction Among American Surgeons. Annals of Surgery. 2009;250(3):463-71. Available from: http://journals.lww.com/annalsofsurgery/Fulltext/2009/09000/Burnout_and_Career_Satisfaction_Among_American.15.aspx.

182. Shanafelt TD, Mungo M, Schmitgen J, Storz KA, Reeves D, Hayes SN, et al., editors. Longitudinal Study Evaluating the Association Between Physician Burnout and Changes in Professional Work Effort. Mayo Clinic Proceedings; 2016: Elsevier. Available from: https://mayoclinic.elsevierpure.com/en/publications/longitudinal-study-evaluating-the-association-between-physician-b

https://carolmilters.com/wp-content/uploads/2022/07/Longitudinal-Study-Evaluating-the-Association-Between-Physician-Burnout-and-Changes-in-Professional-Work-Effort-Mayo-Clinic-2016.pdf.

183. Sokolova O, Pogosova N, Isakova S. Impact of primary care physicians burnout on their adherence to national guidelines for common CVD. Global Heart. 2018;13:486. Available from: https://www.sciencedirect.com/science/article/abs/pii/S2211816018305416.

184. Barnett K, Mercer SW, Norbury M, Watt G, Wyke S, Guthrie B. Epidemiology of multimorbidity and implications for health care, research, and medical education: a cross-sectional study. The Lancet. 2012;380(9836):37-43. Available from: http://www.sciencedirect.com/science/article/pii/S0140673612602402.

185. Disease GBD, Injury I, Prevalence C, Vos T, Allen C, Arora M, et al. Global, regional, and national incidence, prevalence, and years lived with disability for 310 diseases and injuries, 1990–2015: a systematic analysis for the

Global Burden of Disease Study 2015. The Lancet. 2016;388(10053):1545-602. Available from: https://www.thelancet.com/journals/lancet/article/PIIS0140-6736(16)31678-6/fulltext

https://www.thelancet.com/pdfs/journals/lancet/PIIS0140-6736%2816%2931678-6.pdf.

186. Vos T, Barber RM, Bell B, Bertozzi-Villa A, Biryukov S, Bolliger I, et al. Global, regional, and national incidence, prevalence, and years lived with disability for 301 acute and chronic diseases and injuries in 188 countries, 1990-2013: A systematic analysis for the Global Burden of Disease Study 2013. The Lancet. 2015;386(9995):743-800. Available from: https://www.thelancet.com/journals/lancet/article/PIIS0140-6736(15)60692-4/abstract?code=lancet-site&elsca4=Public+Health%7CInfectious+Diseases%7CHealth+Policy%7CInternal%2FFamily+Medicine%7CGeneral+Surgery%7CLancet

https://drive.google.com/file/d/1LsvGdHNwLDGL9opCxzjqYMRM_PH9Pksq/view.

187. Schulz KF, Altman DG, Moher D. CONSORT 2010 statement: updated guidelines for reporting parallel group randomised trials. BMC medicine. 2010;8(1):18. Available from: http://www.biomedcentral.com/content/pdf/1741-7015-8-18.pdf.

188. Jaffe S. US Congress lets Medicare negotiate lower drug prices. The Lancet. 2022;400(10352):551-2. Available from: https://doi.org/10.1016/S0140-6736(22)01574-4.

189. Shih C, Schwartz J, Coukell A. How Would Government Negotiation of Medicare Part D Drug Prices Work? Health Affairs Forefront. 2016. Available from: https://www.healthaffairs.org/content/forefront/would-government-negotiation-medicare-part-d-drug-prices-work.

190. Scholar G. Google Scholar profile of Benjamin Djulbegovic: Google; 2023 [Google Scholar profile of Benjamin Djulbegovic]. Available from: https://scholar.google.com/citations?hl=en&user=NhekIjsAAAAJ.

191. Schnelle C, Jones MA. Characteristics of exceptionally good doctors: A protocol for a cross-sectional survey of adults. Patient Relat Outcome Meas. 2022(13):181-8. Available from: https://www.tandfonline.com/doi/full/10.2147/PROM.S376033

https://www.tandfonline.com/doi/pdf/10.2147/PROM.S376033.

192. Schnelle C, Jones MA. Characteristics of exceptionally good Doctors—A survey of public adults. Heliyon. 2023;9(2):e13115. Available from: https://www.sciencedirect.com/science/article/pii/S2405844023003225.

193. Perlis RH, Ognyanova K, Uslu A, Lunz Trujillo K, Santillana M, Druckman JN, et al. Trust in Physicians and Hospitals During the COVID-19 Pandemic in a 50-State Survey of US Adults. JAMA Network Open. 2024;7(7):e2424984-e. Available from: https://doi.org/10.1001/jamanetworkopen.2024.24984.

194. Cook AF, Arora VM, Rasinski KA, Curlin FA, Yoon JD. The Prevalence of Medical Student Mistreatment and Its Association With Burnout.

Academic Medicine. 2014;89(5). Available from: https://journals.lww. com/academicmedicine/fulltext/2014/05000/the_prevalence_of_medical_ student_mistreatment_and.22.aspx.

195. Liselotte N. Dyrbye, Matthew R. Thomas, F. Stanford Massie, David V Power, Anne Eacker, William Harper, et al. Burnout and Suicidal Ideation among U.S. Medical Students. Annals of Internal Medicine. 2008;149(5):334-41. Available from: https://www.acpjournals.org/doi/ abs/10.7326/0003-4819-149-5-200809020-00008.

196. Dyrbye LN, Thomas MR, Shanafelt TD. Medical Student Distress: Causes, Consequences, and Proposed Solutions. Mayo Clinic Proceedings. 2005;80(12):1613-22. Available from: https://www.sciencedirect.com/ science/article/pii/S0025619611610574.

197. Zhou AY, Panagioti M, Esmail A, Agius R, Van Tongeren M, Bower P. Factors Associated With Burnout and Stress in Trainee Physicians: A Systematic Review and Meta-analysis. JAMA Network Open. 2020;3(8):e2013761-e. Available from: https://doi.org/10.1001/jamanetworkopen.2020.13761.

198. Willcock SM, Daly MG, Tennant CC, Allard BJ. Burnout and psychiatric morbidity in new medical graduates. Medical Journal of Australia. 2004;181(7):357-60. Available from: https://onlinelibrary.wiley.com/doi/ abs/10.5694/j.1326-5377.2004.tb06325.x.

199. Hannan E, Breslin N, Doherty E, McGreal M, Moneley D, Offiah G. Burnout and stress amongst interns in Irish hospitals: contributing factors and potential solutions. Irish Journal of Medical Science (1971 -). 2018;187(2):301-7. Available from: https://doi.org/10.1007/s11845-017-1688-7.

200. Galam E, Komly V, Tourneur AL, Jund J. Burnout among French GPs in training: a cross-sectional study. British Journal of General Practice. 2013;63(608):e217-e24. Available from: https://bjgp.org/content/ bjgp/63/608/e217.full.pdf.

201. Yager J, Feinstein RE. Medical education meets pharma: moving ahead. Acad Psychiatry. 2010;34(2):92-7. Available from: https://www.researchgate. net/profile/Robert-Feinstein/publication/41910346_Medical_Education_ Meets_Pharma_Moving_Ahead/links/0912f503d2fad6dfab000000/ Medical-Education-Meets-Pharma-Moving-Ahead.pdf.

202. Sierles F, Brodkey A, Cleary L, McCurdy FA, Mintz M, Frank J, et al. Relationships between drug company representatives and medical students: medical school policies and attitudes of student affairs deans and third-year medical students. Academic Psychiatry. 2009;33:478-83. Available from: https://link.springer.com/article/10.1176/appi.ap.33.6.478
https://www.researchgate.net/profile/Fredrick-Mccurdy/ publication/40027243_Relationships_Between_Drug_Company_ Representatives_and_Medical_StudentsMedical_School_Policies_and_ Attitudes_of_Student_Affairs_Deans_and_Third-Year_Medical_Students/ links/55bfc61808aed621de13a113/Relationships-Between-Drug-Company-Representatives-and-Medical-StudentsMedical-School-Policies-and-Attitudes-of-Student-Affairs-Deans-and-Third-Year-Medical-Students.pdf.

203. Fred HL. Dishonesty in medicine revisited. Tex Heart Inst J. 2008;35(1):6-15.

204. Bilimoria KY, Chung JW, Hedges LV, Dahlke AR, Love R, Cohen ME, et al. National Cluster-Randomized Trial of Duty-Hour Flexibility in Surgical Training. New England Journal of Medicine. 2016;374(8):713-27. Available from: http://www.nejm.org/doi/full/10.1056/NEJMoa1515724.

205. Starfield B, Shi L, Macinko J. Contribution of Primary Care to Health Systems and Health. The Milbank Quarterly. 2005;83(3):457-502. Available from: https://onlinelibrary.wiley.com/doi/abs/10.1111/j.1468-0009.2005.00409.x.

206. OECD. Life Expectancy at Birth. 2023. Available from: https://www.oecd-ilibrary.org/life-expectancy-at-birth_d90b402d-en.pdf?itemId=%2Fcontent%2Fcomponent%2Fd90b402d-en&mimeType=pdf.

207. Davis LC, Diianni AT, Drumheller SR, Elansary NN, D'Ambrozio GN, Herrawi F, et al. Undisclosed financial conflicts of interest in DSM-5-TR: cross sectional analysis. BMJ. 2024;384:e076902. Available from: https://www.bmj.com/content/bmj/384/bmj-2023-076902.full.pdf.

208. Cosgrove L, Krimsky S. A Comparison of DSM-IV and DSM-5 Panel Members' Financial Associations with Industry: A Pernicious Problem Persists. PLoS Med. 2012;9(3):e1001190. Available from: https://journals.plos.org/plosmedicine/article?id=10.1371/journal.pmed.1001190.

209. Oster G, Thompson D, Edelsberg J, Bird AP, Colditz GA. Lifetime health and economic benefits of weight loss among obese persons. American Journal of Public Health. 1999;89(10):1536-42. Available from: http://www.ncbi.nlm.nih.gov/pmc/articles/PMC1508787/pdf/amjph00010-0078.pdf.

210. Miller NH, Hill M, Kottke T, Ockene IS. The multilevel compliance challenge: Recommendations for a call to action A statement for healthcare professionals. Circulation. 1997;95(4):1085-90. Available from: https://www.ahajournals.org/doi/full/10.1161/01.CIR.95.4.1085.

211. Turk DC, Rudy TE. Neglected topics in the treatment of chronic pain patients—relapse, noncompliance, and adherence enhancement. Pain. 1991;44(1):5-28. Available from: https://journals.lww.com/pain/abstract/1991/01000/neglected_topics_in_the_treatment_of_chronic_pain.3.aspx.

212. Middleton KR, Anton SD, Perri MG. Long-Term Adherence to Health Behavior Change. American Journal of Lifestyle Medicine. 2013;7(6):395-404. Available from: https://journals.sagepub.com/doi/abs/10.1177/1559827613488867.

213. Burgess E, Hassmén P, Pumpa KL. Determinants of adherence to lifestyle intervention in adults with obesity: a systematic review. Clinical Obesity. 2017;7(3):123-35. Available from: https://onlinelibrary.wiley.com/doi/abs/10.1111/cob.12183.

214. Sunanda Creagh, The Conversation. INTERACTIVE: We mapped cancer rates across Australia – search for your postcode here: The Conversation; 2018 [15/9/2018]. Available from: https://theconversation.com/interactive-we-mapped-cancer-rates-across-australia-search-for-your-postcode-here-102256.

215. Margaret Menge. 163% Increase in Deaths of working people ages 18-64 - Life Insurance Policies in 2021 following Covid-19 vaccine mandate

[Website]. vaccineimpact.com; 2022 [June 17th, 2022]. Available from: https://vaccineimpact.com/2022/fifth-largest-life-insurance-company-in-us-paid-out-163-more-for-deaths-of-working-people-ages-18-64-in-2021-after-covid-19-vaccine-mandates/.

216. Kim HJ, Kim M-H, Choi MG, Chun EM. Psychiatric adverse events following COVID-19 vaccination: a population-based cohort study in Seoul, South Korea. Molecular Psychiatry. 2024. Available from: https://doi.org/10.1038/s41380-024-02627-0.

217. Roh JH, Jung I, Suh Y, Kim M-H. A potential association between COVID-19 vaccination and development of alzheimer's disease. QJM: An International Journal of Medicine. 2024. Available from: https://doi.org/10.1093/qjmed/hcae103.

218. Wells CR, Galvani AP. Impact of the COVID-19 pandemic on cancer incidence and mortality. The Lancet Public Health. 2022;7(6):e490-e1. Available from: https://doi.org/10.1016/S2468-2667(22)00111-6.

219. Mintzes B. Evidence-based medicine: strengths and limitations. Australian Prescriber. 2013. Available from: https://www.nps.org.au/australian-prescriber/articles/evidence-based-medicine-strengths-and-limitations.

220. Lundh A, Sismondo S, Lexchin J, Busuioc OA, Bero L. Industry sponsorship and research outcome. The Cochrane Library. 2012. Available from: https://www.cochranelibrary.com/cdsr/doi/10.1002/14651858.MR000033.pub3/full

https://mai68.org/spip2/IMG/pdf/Lundh_et_al-2017-Cochrane_Database_of_Systematic_Reviews.pdf.

221. Angell M. Industry-sponsored clinical research: A broken system. JAMA. 2008;300(9):1069-71. Available from: http://dx.doi.org/10.1001/jama.300.9.1069.

222. Bero LA. Tobacco industry manipulation of research. Public Health Reports. 2005;120(2):200-8. Available from: http://www.ncbi.nlm.nih.gov/pmc/articles/PMC1497700/.

223. (NIH) NIoH. Who We Are. In: Services UDoHaH, editor. 2024. Available from: https://www.nih.gov/about-nih/who-we-are#:~:text=The%20National%20Institutes%20of%20Health,improve%20health%20and%20save%20olives.

224. Wang Y, Zhang D, Du G, Du R, Zhao J, Jin Y, et al. Remdesivir in adults with severe COVID-19: a randomised, double-blind, placebo-controlled, multicentre trial. The Lancet. 2020;395(10236):1569-78. Available from: https://doi.org/10.1016/S0140-6736(20)31022-9.

225. Kofi Ayittey F, Dzuvor C, Kormla Ayittey M, Bennita Chiwero N, Habib A. Updates on Wuhan 2019 novel coronavirus epidemic. J Med Virol. 2020;92(4):403-7. Available from: https://pmc.ncbi.nlm.nih.gov/articles/PMC7167026/.

226. Zhang L, Shen F-m, Chen F, Lin Z. Origin and Evolution of the 2019 Novel Coronavirus. Clinical Infectious Diseases. 2020;71(15):882-3. Available from: https://doi.org/10.1093/cid/ciaa112.

227. Worobey M. Dissecting the early COVID-19 cases in Wuhan. Science. 2021;374(6572):1202-4. Available from: https://www.science.org/doi/abs/10.1126/science.abm4454.

228. Ben Feuerherd. Everything we know about the Wuhan lab that may have unleashed coronavirus. New York Post. 2020. Available from: https://nypost.com/2020/04/16/all-we-know-about-wuhan-lab-that-may-have-unleashed-covid-19/.

229. Xiao B, Xiao L. alternativenarrative.net. 2020. [cited 2024]. Available from: https://www.alternativenarrative.net/2023/06/the-possible-origins-of-2019-ncov.html.

230. Chan A, The New York Times. Why the Pandemic Probably Started in a Lab, in 5 Key Points2024 2024 June 3, 2024]. Available from: https://www.nytimes.com/interactive/2024/06/03/opinion/covid-lab-leak.html.

231. Jones DA. Coronavirus: Factual Fiction or Fictional Facts? Nveo-Natural Volatiles & Essential Oils Journal| Nveo. 2021;8(4):10626-36. Available from: https://www.nveo.org/index.php/journal/article/view/2181

http://www.nveo.org/index.php/journal/article/download/2181/1926.

232. Komesaroff PA, Dwyer DE. The Question of the Origins of COVID-19 and the Ends of Science. Journal of Bioethical Inquiry. 2023. Available from: https://doi.org/10.1007/s11673-023-10303-1.

233. Duignan B. Occam's razor. Encyclopedia Britannica; 2024. Available from: https://www.britannica.com/topic/Occams-razor.

234. Select Subcommittee on the Coronavirus Pandemic Committee on Oversight and Accountability, U.S. House of Representatives. AFTER ACTION REVIEW OF THE COVID-19 PANDEMIC: The Lessons Learned and a Path Forward Washington DC: United States House of Representatives; 2024 December 4th, 2024. Available from: https://oversight.house.gov/wp-content/uploads/2024/12/12.04.2024-SSCP-FINAL-REPORT.pdf

https://x.com/COVIDSelect/status/1863637369972301868.

235. Saxon S, Thorp JA, Viglione D. The COVID-19 Vaccines & Beyond: What the Medical Industrial Complex is NOT Telling Us. 2023. Available from: https://www.thegms.co/publichealth/pubheal-rw-22092202.pdf.

236. Mike Yeadon. Doctors for COVID Ethics [Internet]2022. [cited 2024]. Available from: https://doctors4covidethics.org/the-covid-lies/.

237. Breggin PR, Breggin GR, McCullough PA, Vliet EL. COVID-19 and the Global Predators: Lake Edge Press; 2021. Available from: chrome-extension://efaidnbmnnnibpcajpcglclefindmkaj/https://pearl-hifi.com/11_Spirited_Growth/10_Health_Neg/04_Pandemics/05_COVID_19/Books/COVID-19_and_The_Global_Predators_We_are_the_Prey.pdf.

238. c19 Collective. c19ivm.org Ivermectin for COVID-19: real-time meta analysis of 100 studies 2024 [Available from: https://c19ivm.org/meta.html.

239. Adams MJ, Lefkowitz EJ, King AMQ, Harrach B, Harrison RL, Knowles NJ, et al. 50 years of the International Committee on Taxonomy of Viruses:

progress and prospects. Archives of Virology. 2017;162(5):1441-6. Available from: https://doi.org/10.1007/s00705-016-3215-y.

240. Gillham NW. A life of Sir Francis Galton: From African exploration to the birth of eugenics: Oxford University Press, USA; 2001.

241. Kuhl S. The Nazi connection: Eugenics, American racism, and German national socialism: Oxford University Press; 2002.

242. Garver KL, Garver B. Eugenics: past, present, and the future. Am J Hum Genet. 1991;49(5):1109-18. Available from: https://pmc.ncbi.nlm.nih.gov/articles/PMC1683254/

https://pmc.ncbi.nlm.nih.gov/articles/PMC1683254/pdf/ajhg00082-0206.pdf.

243. Jacobsen A. Operation Paperclip. The Secret Intelligence Program That Brought Nazi Scientists To America. New York: Little, Brown and Company; 2014.

244. Johnson K. A Scientific Method to the Madness of Unit 731's Human Experimentation and Biological Warfare Program. Journal of the History of Medicine and Allied Sciences. 2021;77(1):24-47. Available from: https://doi.org/10.1093/jhmas/jrab044.

245. Dahlquist M, Kugelberg HD. Public justification and expert disagreement over non-pharmaceutical interventions for the COVID-19 pandemic. Journal of Medical Ethics. 2023;49(1):9-13. Available from: https://jme.bmj.com/content/medethics/49/1/9.full.pdf.

246. Azevedo F, Pavlović T, Rêgo GG, Ay FC, Gjoneska B, Etienne TW, et al. Social and moral psychology of COVID-19 across 69 countries. Scientific Data. 2023;10(1):272. Available from: https://doi.org/10.1038/s41597-023-02080-8.

247. Kirkpatrick GL. THE COMMON COLD. Primary Care: Clinics in Office Practice. 1996;23(4):657-75. Available from: https://www.sciencedirect.com/science/article/pii/S0095454305703559.

248. Jiang C, Yao X, Zhao Y, Wu J, Huang P, Pan C, et al. Comparative review of respiratory diseases caused by coronaviruses and influenza A viruses during epidemic season. Microbes and Infection. 2020;22(6):236-44. Available from: https://www.sciencedirect.com/science/article/pii/S1286457920300836.

249. Funck-Brentano C, Salem J-E. RETRACTED: Chloroquine or hydroxychloroquine for COVID-19: why might they be hazardous? The Lancet. 2020. Available from: https://doi.org/10.1016/S0140-6736(20)31174-0.

250. Uk N. Pregnancy, breastfeeding and fertility while taking hydroxychloroquine. In: NHS, editor. 2022. Available from: https://www.nhs.uk/medicines/hydroxychloroquine/pregnancy-breastfeeding-and-fertility-while-taking-hydroxychloroquine/.

251. Kisielinski K, Giboni P, Prescher A, Klosterhalfen B, Graessel D, Funken S, et al. Is a Mask That Covers the Mouth and Nose Free from Undesirable Side Effects in Everyday Use and Free of Potential Hazards? International Journal of Environmental Research and Public Health. 2021;18(8):4344. Available from: https://www.mdpi.com/1660-4601/18/8/4344.

252. Rancourt DG. Review of scientific reports of harms caused by face masks, up to February 2021. February; 2021. Available from: https://covid-unmasked.net/wp-content/uploads/2021/02/5thsciencereview-masksharm-1.pdf.

253. Henning Bundgaard, Johan Skov Bundgaard, Daniel Emil Tadeusz Raaschou-Pedersen, Christian von Buchwald, Tobias Todsen, Jakob Boesgaard Norsk, et al. Effectiveness of Adding a Mask Recommendation to Other Public Health Measures to Prevent SARS-CoV-2 Infection in Danish Mask Wearers. Annals of Internal Medicine. 2021;174(3):335-43. Available from: https://www.acpjournals.org/doi/abs/10.7326/M20-6817.

254. Spinner CD, Gottlieb RL, Criner GJ, Arribas López JR, Cattelan AM, Soriano Viladomiu A, et al. Effect of Remdesivir vs Standard Care on Clinical Status at 11 Days in Patients With Moderate COVID-19: A Randomized Clinical Trial. JAMA. 2020;324(11):1048-57. Available from: https://doi.org/10.1001/jama.2020.16349.

255. Anonymous. c19hcq.org HCQ for COVID-19: real-time meta analysis of 421 studies 2024 [

256. Frontera JA, Rahimian JO, Yaghi S, et al. Treatment with Zinc is Associated with Reduced In-Hospital Mortality Among COVID-19 Patients: A Multi-Center Cohort Study2020 2024. 1-25 p. Available from: https://doi.org/10.21203/rs.3.rs-94509/v1.

257. Derwand R, Scholz M. Does zinc supplementation enhance the clinical efficacy of chloroquine/hydroxychloroquine to win today's battle against COVID-19? Medical Hypotheses. 2020;142:109815. Available from: https://www.sciencedirect.com/science/article/pii/S0306987720306435.

258. c19 Collective. COVID-19 early treatment: real-time analysis of 4,345 studies 2024 [Available from: https://c19early.org/.

259. The RECOVERY Collaborative Group, Peter Horby, Marion Mafham, Louise Linsell, Jennifer L. Bell, Natalie Staplin, et al. Effect of Hydroxychloroquine in Hospitalized Patients with Covid-19. New England Journal of Medicine. 2020;383(21):2030-40. Available from: https://www.nejm.org/doi/full/10.1056/NEJMoa2022926.

260. WHO Solidarity Trial Consortium, Hongchao Pan, Richard Peto, Ana-Maria Henao-Restrepo, Marie-Pierre Preziosi, Vasee Sathiyamoorthy, et al. Repurposed Antiviral Drugs for Covid-19 — Interim WHO Solidarity Trial Results. New England Journal of Medicine. 2021;384(6):497-511. Available from: https://www.nejm.org/doi/full/10.1056/NEJMoa2023184.

261. Axfors C, Schmitt AM, Janiaud P, van't Hooft J, Abd-Elsalam S, Abdo EF, et al. Mortality outcomes with hydroxychloroquine and chloroquine in COVID-19 from an international collaborative meta-analysis of randomized trials. Nature Communications. 2021;12(1):2349. Available from: https://doi.org/10.1038/s41467-021-22446-z.

262. c19 Collective. c19hcq.org discussing "Deaths induced by compassionate use of hydroxychloroquine during the first COVID-19 wave: an estimate" by Pradelle et al. doi:10.1016/j.biopha.2023.116055 2024 [Available from: https://c19hcq.org/pradelle.html.

263. c19 Collective. c19hcq.org discussing "Effect of Hydroxychloroquine in Hospitalized Patients with COVID-19: Preliminary results from a multi-centre, randomized, controlled trial" by the RECOVERY Collaborative Group, doi:10.1056/NEJMoa2022926 2024 [Available from: https://c19hcq.org/recovery.html.

264. Nielsen KFM. Kristian Francisco Milla Nielsen [Internet]: Medium.com. 2021. [cited 2024]. Available from: https://kristianfranciscomillanielsen.medium.com/analysis-of-the-hydroxychloroquine-dosing-regimen-in-recovery-and-solidarity-b45a6b99a041.

265. Zelenko V. Dr. Zelenko's @ZelenkoZev Monumental First Video to President Donald Trump from March 21, 2020: Twitter; 2020 [updated March 21, 2020. Tweet]. Available from: https://x.com/DschlopesIsBack/status/1520105144624558082

https://x.com/DschlopesIsBack/status/1520105865780600832.

266. Elisa Braun, Rym Momtaz. Macron meets with controversial chloroquine doctor touted by Trump. Politico. 2020. Available from: https://www.politico.com/news/2020/04/09/macron-meets-with-controversial-chloroquine-doctor-touted-by-trump-177879.

267. Ioannidis JPA. High-cited favorable studies for COVID-19 treatments ineffective in large trials. Journal of Clinical Epidemiology. 2022;148:1-9. Available from: https://www.sciencedirect.com/science/article/pii/S0895435622000841.

268. Fordham E. The doctor who's curing Covid-19 with zinc and hydroxychloroquine. The Conservative Woman. 2020. Available from: https://www.conservativewoman.co.uk/the-doctor-whos-curing-covid-19-with-hydroxychloroquine/.

269. Just Call Me Jack. Totality of Evidence [Internet]: Totality of Evidence. 2021. [cited 2024]. Available from: https://totalityofevidence.com/hydroxychloroquine/.

270. Nass M. ALLIANCE FOR HUMAN RESEARCH PROTECTION [Internet] 2020. Available from: https://ahrp.org/how-a-false-hydroxychloroquine-narrative-was-created/.

271. Heres S, Davis J, Maino K, Jetzinger E, Kissling W, Leucht S. Why Olanzapine Beats Risperidone, Risperidone Beats Quetiapine, and Quetiapine Beats Olanzapine: An Exploratory Analysis of Head-to-Head Comparison Studies of Second-Generation Antipsychotics. American Journal of Psychiatry. 2006;163(2):185-94. Available from: http://ajp.psychiatryonline.org/doi/abs/10.1176/appi.ajp.163.2.185.

272. Ioannidis JP. The totality of the evidence. Boston Review. 2020;26:22-30. Available from: http://www.zambakari.org/uploads/8/4/8/9/84899028/2_the_totality_of_the_evidence_1.pdf.

273. Rachel Schraer, Jack Goodman. Ivermectin: How false science created a Covid 'miracle' drug. BBC Verify (fact check). BBC2021. Available from: https://www.bbc.com/news/health-58170809.

274. Andrzejewski A. Open The Books [Internet]: Substack. 2024. [cited 2024]. Available from: https://openthebooks.substack.com/p/breaking-big-pharma-paid-690-million.

275. Kory P. Pierre Kory's Medical Musings [Internet]: Pierre Kory. 2022. [cited 2022]. Available from: https://pierrekorymedicalmusings.com/p/the-criminal-censorship-of-ivermectin.

276. Hayward G, Yu L-M, Little P, Gbinigie O, Shanyinde M, Harris V, et al. Ivermectin for COVID-19 in adults in the community (PRINCIPLE): an open, randomised, controlled, adaptive platform trial of short- and longer-term outcomes. Journal of Infection. 2024. Available from: https://doi.org/10.1016/j.jinf.2024.106130.

277. Katz AJ. Here's the Median Age of the Typical Cable News Viewer [August 7]. 2023 [updated 2024. Available from: https://www.adweek.com/tvnewser/heres-the-median-age-of-the-typical-cable-news-viewer/#:~:text=According%20to%20Nielsen%20Live%20%2B7%2Dday,and%20Fox%20News%E2%80%99s%20was%2066.

278. dallasvnn. Miracle Drug? Everything They Don't Want You to Know About Ivermectin2023 February 22, 2024. Available from: https://vigilantnews.com/post/miracle-drug-everything-they-dont-want-you-to-know-about-ivermectin/.

279. Santin AD, Scheim DE, McCullough PA, Yagisawa M, Borody TJ. Ivermectin: a multifaceted drug of Nobel prize-honoured distinction with indicated efficacy against a new global scourge, COVID-19. New Microbes New Infect. 2021;43:100924. Available from: https://pubmed.ncbi.nlm.nih.gov/34466270/.

280. Ndyomugyenyi R, Kabatereine N, Olsen A, Magnussen P. Efficacy of ivermectin and albendazole alone and in combination for treatment of soil-transmitted helminths in pregnancy and adverse events: a randomized open label controlled intervention trial in Masindi district, western Uganda. The American journal of tropical medicine and hygiene. 2008;79(6):856-63. Available from: https://www.researchgate.net/profile/Pascal-Magnussen/publication/23567237_Efficacy_of_Ivermectin_and_Albendazole_Alone_and_in_Combination_for_Treatment_of_Soil-Transmitted_Helminths_in_Pregnancy_and_Adverse_Events_A_Randomized_Open_Label_Controlled_Intervention_Trial_in_Mas/links/0a85e537dec804ca04000000/Efficacy-of-Ivermectin-and-Albendazole-Alone-and-in-Combination-for-Treatment-of-Soil-Transmitted-Helminths-in-Pregnancy-and-Adverse-Events-A-Randomized-Open-Label-Controlled-Intervention-Trial-in-Mas.pdf.

281. Õmura S, Crump A. The life and times of ivermectin — a success story. Nature Reviews Microbiology. 2004;2(12):984-9. Available from: https://doi.org/10.1038/nrmicro1048.

282. Laing R, Gillan V, Devaney E. Ivermectin; Old Drug, New Tricks? Trends in Parasitology. 2017;33(6):463-72. Available from: https://doi.org/10.1016/j.pt.2017.02.004.

283. Tang M, Hu X, Wang Y, Yao X, Zhang W, Yu C, et al. Ivermectin, a potential anticancer drug derived from an antiparasitic drug. Pharmacological Research. 2021;163:105207. Available from: https://www.sciencedirect.com/science/article/pii/S1043661820315152.

284. Chen L, Bi S, Wei Q, Zhao Z, Wang C, Xie S. Ivermectin suppresses tumour growth and metastasis through degradation of PAK1 in oesophageal squamous cell carcinoma. Journal of Cellular and Molecular Medicine. 2020;24(9):5387-401. Available from: https://onlinelibrary.wiley.com/doi/abs/10.1111/jcmm.15195.

285. Lee DE, Kang HW, Kim SY, Kim MJ, Jeong JW, Hong WC, et al. Ivermectin and gemcitabine combination treatment induces apoptosis of pancreatic cancer cells via mitochondrial dysfunction. Front Pharmacol. 2022;13:934746. Available from: https://www.frontiersin.org/journals/pharmacology/articles/10.3389/fphar.2022.934746/full

https://www.frontiersin.org/journals/pharmacology/articles/10.3389/fphar.2022.934746/pdf.

286. Li N, Zhan X. Anti-parasite drug ivermectin can suppress ovarian cancer by regulating lncRNA-EIF4A3-mRNA axes. Epma j. 2020;11(2):289-309. Available from: https://link.springer.com/article/10.1007/s13167-020-00209-y

https://link.springer.com/content/pdf/10.1007/s13167-020-00209-y.pdf.

287. Zhou S, Wu H, Ning W, Wu X, Xu X, Ma Y, et al. Ivermectin has New Application in Inhibiting Colorectal Cancer Cell Growth. Frontiers in Pharmacology. 2021;12. Available from: https://www.frontiersin.org/articles/10.3389/fphar.2021.717529.

288. Draganov D, Han Z, Rana A, Bennett N, Irvine DJ, Lee PP. Ivermectin converts cold tumors hot and synergizes with immune checkpoint blockade for treatment of breast cancer. npj Breast Cancer. 2021;7(1):22. Available from: https://doi.org/10.1038/s41523-021-00229-5.

289. Jiang L, Wang P, Sun YJ, Wu YJ. Ivermectin reverses the drug resistance in cancer cells through EGFR/ERK/Akt/NF-κB pathway. J Exp Clin Cancer Res. 2019;38(1):265. Available from: https://link.springer.com/article/10.1186/s13046-019-1251-7

https://link.springer.com/content/pdf/10.1186/s13046-019-1251-7.pdf.

290. Guzzo CA, Furtek CI, Porras AG, Chen C, Tipping R, Clineschmidt CM, et al. Safety, Tolerability, and Pharmacokinetics of Escalating High Doses of Ivermectin in Healthy Adult Subjects. The Journal of Clinical Pharmacology. 2002;42(10):1122-33. Available from: https://accp1.onlinelibrary.wiley.com/doi/abs/10.1177/009127002237994.

291. Grace PA. Therapeutic bloodletting in Ireland from the medieval period to modern times. Proceedings of the Royal Irish Academy: Archaeology, Culture, History, Literature. 2021;121(1):227-48. Available from: https://muse.jhu.edu/view_citations?type=article&id=838623.

292. Firdaus SU. The urgency of legal regulations existence in case of COVID-19 vaccination refusal in Indonesia. Journal of Forensic and Legal Medicine.

2022;91:102401. Available from: https://www.sciencedirect.com/science/article/pii/S1752928X22000993.

293. Figueroa JP, Bottazzi ME, Hotez P, Batista C, Ergonul O, Gilbert S, et al. Urgent needs of low-income and middle-income countries for COVID-19 vaccines and therapeutics. The Lancet. 2021;397(10274):562-4. Available from: https://doi.org/10.1016/S0140-6736(21)00242-7.

294. Schmidt H. Vaccine Rationing and the Urgency of Social Justice in the Covid-19 Response. Hastings Center Report. 2020;50(3):46-9. Available from: https://onlinelibrary.wiley.com/doi/abs/10.1002/hast.1113.

295. Burgos RM, Badowski ME, Drwiega E, Ghassemi S, Griffith N, Herald F, et al. The race to a COVID-19 vaccine: opportunities and challenges in development and distribution. Drugs Context. 2021;10. Available from: https://pmc.ncbi.nlm.nih.gov/articles/PMC7889064/

https://pdfs.semanticscholar.org/5fb8/15b401453df7bd77e4a1c287b441abe2b186.pdf.

296. Collins FS, Stoffels P. Accelerating COVID-19 Therapeutic Interventions and Vaccines (ACTIV): An Unprecedented Partnership for Unprecedented Times. JAMA. 2020;323(24):2455-7. Available from: https://doi.org/10.1001/jama.2020.8920.

297. Ferdinands JM, Rao S, Dixon BE, Mitchell PK, DeSilva MB, Irving SA, et al. Waning 2-Dose and 3-Dose Effectiveness of mRNA Vaccines Against COVID-19-Associated Emergency Department and Urgent Care Encounters and Hospitalizations Among Adults During Periods of Delta and Omicron Variant Predominance - VISION Network, 10 States, August 2021-January 2022. MMWR Morb Mortal Wkly Rep. 2022;71(7):255-63. Available from: https://www.cdc.gov/mmwr/volumes/71/wr/mm7107e2.htm?utm_source=miragenews&utm_medium=miragenews&utm_campaign=news.

298. Lamb YN. BNT162b2 mRNA COVID-19 Vaccine: First Approval. Drugs. 2021;81(4):495-501. Available from: https://doi.org/10.1007/s40265-021-01480-7.

299. Fortner A, Schumacher D. First COVID-19 Vaccines Receiving the US FDA and EMA Emergency Use Authorization. Discoveries (Craiova). 2021;9(1):e122. Available from: https://pmc.ncbi.nlm.nih.gov/articles/PMC8101362/.

300. Iwry JL. FDA Emergency Use Authorization From 9/11 to COVID-19: Historical Lessons and Ethical Challenges. Food & Drug LJ. 2021;76:337. Available from: https://heinonline.org/HOL/LandingPage?handle=hein.journals/foodlj76&div=17&id=&page=

https://papers.ssrn.com/sol3/Delivery.cfm?abstractid=3902890.

301. Bramante CT, Huling JD, Tignanelli CJ, Buse JB, Liebovitz DM, Nicklas JM, et al. Randomized Trial of Metformin, Ivermectin, and Fluvoxamine for Covid-19. New England Journal of Medicine. 2022;387(7):599-610. Available from: https://www.nejm.org/doi/full/10.1056/NEJMoa2201662.

302. Naggie S, Boulware DR, Lindsell CJ, Stewart TG, Gentile N, Collins S, et al. Effect of Ivermectin vs Placebo on Time to Sustained Recovery in Outpatients With Mild to Moderate COVID-19: A Randomized Clinical

Trial. JAMA. 2022;328(16):1595-603. Available from: https://doi.org/10.1001/jama.2022.18590.

303. Kory P. Pierre Kory's Medical Musings [Internet]: Pierre Kory. 2022. [cited 2022]. Available from: https://pierrekorymedicalmusings.com/p/the-publication-of-fraudulent-ivermectin-da1.

304. Kory P. Pierre Kory Medical Musings [Internet]2022. [cited 2024]. Available from: https://pierrekorymedicalmusings.com/p/the-publication-of-fraudulent-ivermectin-da1.

305. Kory P. Pierre Kory Medical Musings [Internet]2022 2024. Available from: https://pierrekorymedicalmusings.com/p/the-publication-of-fraudulent-ivermectin.

306. Kory P. Pierre Kory Medical Musings [Internet]2022 2024. [cited 2024]. Available from: https://pierrekorymedicalmusings.com/p/the-criminal-censorship-of-ivermectin.

307. Edmund J Fordham, Theresa A Lawrie, Katherine McGilchrist, Andrew Bryant. The uses and abuses of systematic reviews: the case of ivermectin in Covid-19. Available from: https://osf.io/preprints/osf/mp4f2.

308. Alexander S. Astral Codex Ten [Internet]2023. Available from: https://www.astralcodexten.com/p/ivermectin-much-more-than-you-wanted.

309. Pablo, Michael A, Ryan Carey, Leo. Effective Altruism Forum [Internet]: effectivealtruism.com. 2022. Available from: https://forum.effectivealtruism.org/topics/scott-alexander

https://lorienpsych.com/about/

https://www.astralcodexten.com/about.

310. Marinos A. Do Your Own Research [Internet]: Substack. 2022. [cited 2024]. Available from: https://doyourownresearch.substack.com/p/the-potemkin-argument-index.

311. Marinos A. Do Your Own Research [Internet]: Substack. 2022. [cited 2024]. Available from: https://doyourownresearch.substack.com/p/the-potemkin-argument-index.

312. Alexander S. Astral Codex Ten [Internet]2021.

313. Adam D. The data detective. Nature. 2019;571(7766):462-4. Available from: https://www.nature.com/articles/d41586-019-02241-z.

314. Bitterman A, Martins CP, Cices A, Nadendla MP. Comparison of Trials Using Ivermectin for COVID-19 Between Regions With High and Low Prevalence of Strongyloidiasis: A Meta-analysis. JAMA Network Open. 2022;5(3):e223079-e. Available from: https://doi.org/10.1001/jamanetworkopen.2022.3079.

315. Marinos A. Do Your Own Research [Internet]: Substack. 2022. [cited 2024]. Available from: https://doyourownresearch.substack.com/p/the-potemkin-argument-index.

316. Costa-Cruz JM, Paula FM. Epidemiological aspects of strongyloidiasis in Brazil. Parasitology. 2011;138(11):1331-40. Available from: https://www.cambridge.org/core/product/F2F1D0B595902E19DBF65DCB3809D7FC.

317. Buonfrate D, Bisanzio D, Giorli G, Odermatt P, Fürst T, Greenaway C, et al. The Global Prevalence of Strongyloides stercoralis Infection. Pathogens. 2020;9(6):468. Available from: https://www.mdpi.com/2076-0817/9/6/468.

318. Merck Staff Writer. Merck Statement on Ivermectin use During the COVID-19 Pandemic: Merck; 2021 [Available from: https://www.merck.com/news/merck-statement-on-ivermectin-use-during-the-covid-19-pandemic/#.

319. HCCA SW. CMS Hikes Payment for COVID-19 Inpatients Treated With New Drugs, Links it to 20% Bonus (Remdesivir and Covid-19 convalescent plasma). 2020. Available from: https://www.jdsupra.com/legalnews/cms-hikes-payment-for-covid-19-19452/.

320. Ioannidis J. The infection fatality rate of COVID-19 inferred from seroprevalence data (preprint). 2020. Available from: https://pmc.ncbi.nlm.nih.gov/articles/PMC7947934/

https://biomechanics.stanford.edu/me233_20/reading/ioannidis20.pdf.

321. Pezzullo AM, Axfors C, Contopoulos-Ioannidis DG, Apostolatos A, Ioannidis JPA. Age-stratified infection fatality rate of COVID-19 in the non-elderly population. Environmental Research. 2023;216:114655. Available from: https://www.sciencedirect.com/science/article/pii/S001393512201982X.

322. Lu Y, Wang Y, Shen C, Luo J, Yu W. Decreased Incidence of Influenza During the COVID-19 Pandemic. International Journal of General Medicine. 2022;15(null):2957-62. Available from: https://www.tandfonline.com/doi/abs/10.2147/IJGM.S343940.

323. Agca H, Akalin H, Saglik I, Hacimustafaoglu M, Celebi S, Ener B. Changing epidemiology of influenza and other respiratory viruses in the first year of COVID-19 pandemic. Journal of Infection and Public Health. 2021;14(9):1186-90. Available from: https://www.sciencedirect.com/science/article/pii/S1876034121002227.

324. Olsen SJ, Winn AK, Budd AP, Prill MM, Steel J, Midgley CM, et al. Changes in Influenza and Other Respiratory Virus Activity During the COVID-19 Pandemic - United States, 2020-2021. MMWR Morb Mortal Wkly Rep. 2021;70(29):1013-9. Available from: https://www.cdc.gov/mmwr/volumes/70/wr/mm7029a1.htm.

325. Solomon DA, Sherman AC, Kanjilal S. Influenza in the COVID-19 Era. JAMA. 2020;324(13):1342-3. Available from: https://doi.org/10.1001/jama.2020.14661.

326. Li P, Wang Y, Peppelenbosch MP, Ma Z, Pan Q. Systematically comparing COVID-19 with the 2009 influenza pandemic for hospitalized patients. International Journal of Infectious Diseases. 2021;102:375-80. Available from: https://www.sciencedirect.com/science/article/pii/S1201971220323213.

327. Andrew MK, MacDonald S, Ye L, Ambrose A, Boivin G, Diaz-Mitoma F, et al. Impact of Frailty on Influenza Vaccine Effectiveness and Clinical Outcomes: Experience From the Canadian Immunization Research Network (CIRN) Serious Outcomes Surveillance (SOS) Network 2011/12 Season. Open Forum Infectious Diseases. 2016;3(suppl_1). Available from: https://doi.org/10.1093/ofid/ofw172.573.

328. Schaffner W, McElhaney J, Rizzo AA, Savoy M, Taylor AJ, Young M. The Dangers of Influenza and Benefits of Vaccination in Adults With Chronic Health Conditions. Infectious Diseases in Clinical Practice. 2018;26(6). Available from: https://journals.lww.com/infectdis/fulltext/2018/11000/the_dangers_of_influenza_and_benefits_of.3.aspx.

329. Paget J, Spreeuwenberg P, Charu V, Taylor RJ, Iuliano AD, Bresee J, et al. Global mortality associated with seasonal influenza epidemics: New burden estimates and predictors from the GLaMOR Project. J Glob Health. 2019;9(2):020421. Available from: https://pmc.ncbi.nlm.nih.gov/articles/PMC6815659/.

330. Bergman P, Lindh ÅU, Björkhem-Bergman L, Lindh JD. Vitamin D and Respiratory Tract Infections: A Systematic Review and Meta-Analysis of Randomized Controlled Trials. PLOS ONE. 2013;8(6):e65835. Available from: https://doi.org/10.1371/journal.pone.0065835.

331. Jolliffe DA, Camargo CA, Jr., Sluyter JD, Aglipay M, Aloia JF, Ganmaa D, et al. Vitamin D supplementation to prevent acute respiratory infections: a systematic review and meta-analysis of aggregate data from randomised controlled trials. The Lancet Diabetes & Endocrinology. 2021;9(5):276-92. Available from: https://doi.org/10.1016/S2213-8587(21)00051-6.

332. Teshome A, Adane A, Girma B, Mekonnen ZA. The Impact of Vitamin D Level on COVID-19 Infection: Systematic Review and Meta-Analysis. Frontiers in Public Health. 2021;9. Available from: https://www.frontiersin.org/journals/public-health/articles/10.3389/fpubh.2021.624559.

333. Ganmaa D, Enkhmaa D, Nasantogtokh E, Sukhbaatar S, Tumur-Ochir K-E, Manson J. Vitamin D, respiratory infections, and chronic disease: Review of meta-analyses and randomized clinical trials. Journal of Internal Medicine. 2022;291(2):141-64. Available from: https://onlinelibrary.wiley.com/doi/abs/10.1111/joim.13399

https://onlinelibrary.wiley.com/doi/pdfdirect/10.1111/joim.13399?download=true.

334. Jefferson T, Heneghan C. Trust the Evidence [Internet]: Substack. 2024. [cited 2024]. Available from: https://trusttheevidence.substack.com/p/a-roundup-of-the-story-of-cochrane.

335. Soares-Weiser K, Lasserson T, Jorgensen KJ, Woloshin S, Bero L, Brown MD, et al. Policy makers must act on incomplete evidence in responding to COVID-19. Cochrane Database of Systematic Reviews. 2020(11). Available from: https://doi.org//10.1002/14651858.ED000149.

336. McNaughton CD, Adams NM, Hirschie Johnson C, Ward MJ, Schmitz JE, Lasko TA. Diurnal Variation in SARS-CoV-2 PCR Test Results: Test Accuracy May Vary by Time of Day. Journal of Biological Rhythms. 2021;36(6):595-601. Available from: https://journals.sagepub.com/doi/abs/10.1177/07487304211051841.

337. Khullar D, Bond AM, Schpero WL. COVID-19 and the Financial Health of US Hospitals. JAMA. 2020;323(21):2127-8. Available from: https://doi.org/10.1001/jama.2020.6269.

338. Ethan Covey. Infectious Disease Special Edition [Internet]2021. [cited 2024]. Available from: https://www.idse.net/Covid-19/Article/08-21/ MDs-Spreading-COVID-Vaccine-Misinformation-Risk-Losing-Medical-Licenses/64365.

339. Bay v Australian Health Practitioner Regulation Agency [2024] QSC 315 (2024). Available from: https://archive.sclqld.org.au/qjudgment/2024/ QSC24-315.pdf.

340. Rancourt DG, Baudin M, Hickey J, Mercier J. COVID-19 vaccine-associated mortality in the Southern Hemisphere. CORRELATION Research in the Public Interest. 2023. Available from: https://www.truth11.com/ untitled-1257/.

341. Gibo M, Kojima S, Fujisawa A, Kikuchi T, Fukushima M. Increased Age-Adjusted Cancer Mortality After the Third mRNA-Lipid Nanoparticle Vaccine Dose During the COVID-19 Pandemic in Japan. Cureus. 2024;16(4):e57860. Available from: http://dx.doi.org/10.7759/cureus.57860.

342. Gøtzsche P. Mad in America [Internet]2024. [cited 2024]. Available from: https://www.madinamerica.com/2024/04/prescription-drugs-are-the-leading-cause-of-death/

https://brownstone.org/articles/prescription-drugs-are-the-leading-cause-of-death/.

343. Seidelman WE. The professional origins of Dr. Joseph Mengele. Canadian Medical Association Journal. 1985;133(11):1169-71. Available from: https:// pmc.ncbi.nlm.nih.gov/articles/PMC1346379/

https://pmc.ncbi.nlm.nih.gov/articles/PMC1346379/pdf/canmedaj 00274-0072.pdf.

344. Smith D. Not by Error, But by Design - Harold Shipman and the Regulatory Crisis for Health Care. Public policy and administration. 2002;17(4):55-74. Available from: https://journals.sagepub.com/doi/abs/10.1177/095207670201700405

https://citeseerx.ist.psu.edu/document?repid=rep1&type=pdf&doi=1d9 6871e38eefef5288c1f9dcdf6469f8a89beb4.

345. Dyer C. Investigators should be trained to "think dirty" about cause of death, Shipman report says. BMJ. 2003;327(7407):123. Available from: https://www.bmj.com/content/bmj/327/7407/123.4.full.pdf.

346. Brody H. Hooked: Ethics, the medical profession, and the pharmaceutical industry: Soc Nuclear Med; 2008. Available from: https://web.archive.org/ web/20180720151554id_/http://jnm.snmjournals.org/content/49/12/2068. full.pdf.

347. Rennie D. When evidence isn't: trials, drug companies and the FDA. JL & Pol'y. 2007;15:991. Available from: https://heinonline.org/HOL/ LandingPage?handle=hein.journals/jlawp15&div=37&id=&page=

https://brooklynworks.brooklaw.edu/cgi/viewcontent.cgi?article= 1206&context=jlp.

348. Mundy A. Dispensing with the truth: The victims, the drug companies, and the dramatic story behind the battle over Fen-Phen: St. Martin's Press; 2010.

349. Braithwaite J. Corporate crime in the pharmaceutical industry (Routledge Revivals): Routledge; 2013.

350. Willman D. How a new policy led to seven deadly drugs. Los Angeles Times. 2000;20:1. Available from: https://www.latimes.com/nation/la-122001fda-story.html.

351. Ross DB. The FDA and the case of Ketek. New England Journal of Medicine. 2007;356(16):1601-4. Available from: https://www.nejm.org/doi/full/10.1056/NEJMp078032

https://www.nejm.org/doi/pdf/10.1056/NEJMp078032.

352. Abraham J. Science, politics and the pharmaceutical industry: Controversy and bias in drug regulation: Routledge; 2023.

353. Rosenberg M. Former FDA reviewer speaks out about intimidation, retaliation and marginalizing of safety. Truthout. 2012 29 July 2012. Available from: https://truthout.org/articles/former-fda-reviewer-speaks-out-about-intimidation-retaliation-and-marginalizing-of-safety/.

354. Weingart NS, Wilson RM, Gibberd RW, Harrison B. Epidemiology of medical error. Bmj. 2000;320(7237):774-7. Available from: https://www.ncbi.nlm.nih.gov/pmc/articles/PMC1117772/pdf/774.pdf.

355. Starfield B. Is US health really the best in the world? Jama. 2000;284(4):483-5. Available from: https://jamanetwork.com/journals/jama/article-abstract/192908.

356. Ebbesen J, Buajordet I, Erikssen J, Brørs O, Hilberg T, Svaar H, et al. Drug-related deaths in a department of internal medicine. Archives of internal medicine. 2001;161(19):2317-23. Available from: https://jamanetwork.com/journals/jamainternalmedicine/fullarticle/649279.

357. Kragh A. Two of three people in nursing homes are in treatment with at least ten drugs. Läkartidningen; 2004. Available from: https://pubmed.ncbi.nlm.nih.gov/15055120/

https://www.researchgate.net/publication/8646344_Two_out_of_three_persons_living_in_nursing_homes_for_the_elderly_are_treated_with_at_least_ten_different_drugs_A_survey_of_drug_prescriptions_in_the_northeastern_part_of_Skane.

358. Garfinkel D, Mangin D. Feasibility study of a systematic approach for discontinuation of multiple medications in older adults: addressing polypharmacy. Archives of internal medicine. 2010;170(18):1648-54. Available from: https://jamanetwork.com/journals/jamainternalmedicine/fullarticle/226051.

359. Petersen M. Suit says company promoted drug in exam rooms. The New York Times. 2002 May 15, 2002. Available from: https://www.nytimes.com/2002/05/15/business/suit-says-company-promoted-drug-in-exam-rooms.html.

360. Harris G. Pfizer to pay $430 million over promoting drug to doctors. The New York Times on the Web. 2004 May 14, 2004. Available from: https://www.nytimes.com/2004/05/14/business/pfizer-to-pay-430-million-over-promoting-drug-to-doctors.html.

361. Adams C, Young A. Off-label prescription case reflects federal concern over unsafe uses. Knight Ridder Newspapers. 2004 November 2-4, 2003. Available from: https://www.anderson.ucla.edu/documents/areas/adm/loeb/04h17riskyrx.pdf.

362. Van Voris R, Lawrence J. Pfizer told to pay $142.1 million for Neurontin marketing fraud. Bloomberg News. 2010. Available from: https://www.bloomberg.com/news/articles/2010-02-22/pfizer-begins-trial-of-300-million-neurontin-claim-of-misuse-by-kaiser.

363. Graham DJ. COX-2 inhibitors, other NSAIDs, and cardiovascular risk: the seduction of common sense. Jama. 2006;296(13):1653-6. Available from: https://jamanetwork.com/journals/jama/article-abstract/203465.

364. Psaty BM, Furberg CD. COX-2 inhibitors--lessons in drug safety. New England journal of medicine. 2005;352(11):1133-4. Available from: https://www.nejm.org/doi/abs/10.1056/NEJMe058042

https://www.researchgate.net/profile/Curt-Furberg/publication/8019135_COX-2_Inhibitors_-_Lessons_in_Drug_Safety/links/02e7e52f233b429d1f000000/COX-2-Inhibitors-Lessons-in-Drug-Safety.pdf.

365. Topol EJ. Failing the public health—rofecoxib, Merck, and the FDA. New England Journal of Medicine. 2004;351(17):1707-9. Available from: https://www.nejm.org/doi/full/10.1056/NEJMp048286

https://www.nejm.org/doi/pdf/10.1056/NEJMp048286.

366. Schwartz LM, Woloshin S. How the FDA forgot the evidence: the case of donepezil 23 mg. BMJ. 2012;344. Available from: https://www.bmj.com/content/344/bmj.e1086.long.

367. Lenzer J. FDA is criticised for licensing high dose donepezil. BMJ. 2011;342:d3270. Available from: https://www.bmj.com/content/bmj/342/bmj.d3270.full.pdf.

368. Healy D. Let Them Eat Prozac:

The Unhealthy Relationship Between the Pharmaceutical Industry and Depression. New York: New York University Press; 2024.

369. Caplan PJ. They say you're crazy: How the world's most powerful psychiatrists decide who's normal: Addison-Wesley/Addison Wesley Longman; 1995.

370. Nielsen M, Hansen EH, Gøtzsche PC. What is the difference between dependence and withdrawal reactions? A comparison of benzodiazepines and selective serotonin re-uptake inhibitors. Addiction. 2012;107(5):900-8. Available from: https://onlinelibrary.wiley.com/doi/abs/10.1111/j.1360-0443.2011.03686.x

https://www.researchgate.net/profile/Logan-Netzer/post/Grouping-outcomes-in-meta-analysis-and-change-of-point-estimate-effect-size-Which-one-is-the-correct-Grouping-Not-grouping/attachment/59d63 91679197b80779964d8/AS%3A400376466558978%401472468596941/download/Nielsen+et+al.%2C+2011+withdrawal+-NEED.pdf.

371. Montejo AL, Llorca G, Izquierdo JA, Rico-Villademoros F. Incidence of sexual dysfunction associated with antidepressant agents: a prospective multicenter

study of 1022 outpatients. Journal of Clinical Psychiatry. 2001;62:10-21. Available from: https://www.psychiatrist.com/read-pdf/8888/.

372. 2024. Ether (noun). Available from: https://www.oed.com/dictionary/ether_n?tl=true.

373. Editors Hc. Ether and Chloroform [August 7]. 2024 [updated 2024. Available from: https://www.history.com/topics/inventions/ether-and-chloroform.

374. Bacon DR. Romance, Poetry, and Surgical Sleep: Literature Influences Medicine (review) Johns Hopkins University Press 1996. Available from: https://muse.jhu.edu/pub/1/article/3778

375. University of Bristol SoC. Diethyl Ether [August 7]. 2024 [updated 2024. Available from: https://www.chm.bris.ac.uk/motm/diethyl-ether/etherh.htm.

376. Birkmeyer JD, Reames BN, McCulloch P, Carr AJ, Campbell WB, Wennberg JE. Understanding of regional variation in the use of surgery. The Lancet. 2013;382(9898):1121-9. Available from: https://www.thelancet.com/journals/lancet/article/PIIS0140-6736(13)61215-5/abstract

https://pmc.ncbi.nlm.nih.gov/articles/PMC4211114/.

377. Maurer H. The MD's are off their pedestal. Fortune, Feb. 1954:138-86. Available from: https://ccat.sas.upenn.edu/goldenage/exp/ex_p2_24.htm.

378. Himmelstein DU, Woolhandler S. The Current and Projected Taxpayer Shares of US Health Costs. American Journal of Public Health. 2016;106(3):449-52. Available from: https://ajph.aphapublications.org/doi/abs/10.2105/AJPH.2015.302997.

379. Mary Johnson. Should Congress Limit Health Insurance Company Profits? : seniorsleague.org; 2018 [Available from: https://seniorsleague.org/congress-limit-health-insurance-company-profits/.

380. Staff writer CfMMS. 80/20 Rule Delivers More Value to Consumers in 2012: cms.gov Centers for Medicare & Medicaid Services; 2012 [Available from: https://www.cms.gov/CCIIO/Resources/Forms-Reports-and-Other-Resources/Downloads/2012-medical-loss-ratio-report.pdf.

381. Maulitz RC, Long DE. Grand rounds: One hundred years of internal medicine Beeson and Maulitz "The Inner History of Internal Medicine": University of Pennsylvania Press; 2016.

382. Dowling HF. Fighting infection: conquests of the twentieth century: Harvard University Press; 1977.

383. Starr P. The social transformation of American medicine: Basic Books New York; 1978.

384. Beeson PB, Maulitz RC. The inner history of internal medicine Personal communication from James Wyngaarden cited by Benson and Maulitz 29-30 in the book Grand Rounds by Maulitz and Long1988. 15-54 p. Available from: https://www.degruyter.com/document/doi/10.9783/9781512804294-006/pdf?licenseType=restricted.

385. Leape LL. The Government Responds: The Agency for Healthcare Research and Quality. Making Healthcare Safe: The Story of the Patient Safety Movement. Cham: Springer International Publishing; 2021. p. 143-58. Available from: https://doi.org/10.1007/978-3-030-71123-8_10.

386. Lewis M. The undoing project: A friendship that changed our minds: WW Norton & Company; 2016.

387. Scott IA, Hilmer SN, Reeve E, Potter K, Le Couteur D, Rigby D, et al. Reducing Inappropriate Polypharmacy: The Process of Deprescribing. JAMA Internal Medicine. 2015;175(5):827-34. Available from: https://doi.org/10.1001/jamainternmed.2015.0324.

388. McLeod PJ, Huang AR, Tamblyn RM, Gayton DC. Defining inappropriate practices in prescribing for elderly people: a national consensus panel. Canadian Medical Association Journal. 1997;156(3):385-91. Available from: https://www.cmaj.ca/content/cmaj/156/3/385.full.pdf.

389. McGlynn EA, Asch SM, Adams J, Keesey J, Hicks J, DeCristofaro A, et al. The quality of health care delivered to adults in the United States. New England journal of medicine. 2003;348(26):2635-45. Available from: https://www.nejm.org/doi/full/10.1056/NEJMsa022615

https://www.qualityhealth.org/downloads/scoap/TheQualityof-HealthCare-NEJM.pdf.

390. Rathert C, Williams ES, Linhart H. Evidence for the Quadruple Aim: A Systematic Review of the Literature on Physician Burnout and Patient Outcomes. Med Care. 2018;56(12):976-84. Available from: https://journals.lww.com/lww-medicalcare/abstract/2018/12000/evidence_for_the_quadruple_aim__a_systematic.3.aspx

https://www.ingentaconnect.com/content/wk/mcar/2018/00000056/00000012/art00005%3bjsessionid=sot205atmk8g.x-ic-live-01.

391. Salyers MP, Bonfils KA, Luther L, Firmin RL, White DA, Adams EL, et al. The Relationship Between Professional Burnout and Quality and Safety in Healthcare: A Meta-Analysis. J Gen Intern Med. 2017;32(4):475-82. Available from: https://link.springer.com/article/10.1007/s11606-016-3886-9

https://www.ncbi.nlm.nih.gov/pmc/articles/PMC5377877/pdf/11606_2016_Article_3886.pdf.

392. Wyer P, Alves da Silva S. 'All the King's horses …': the problematical fate of born-again evidence-based medicine: commentary on Greenhalgh, T., Snow, R., Ryan, S., Rees, S., and Salisbury, H. (2015) six 'biases' against patients and carers in evidence-based medicine. BioMed Central Medicine, 13:200. Journal of Evaluation in Clinical Practice. 2015;21(6):E1-E10. Available from: http://dx.doi.org/10.1111/jep.12492.

393. Tovey D, Churchill R, Bero L. Evidence based medicine: looking forward and building on what we have learnt. BMJ. 2014;349. Available from: http://www.bmj.com/content/bmj/349/bmj.g4508.full.pdf.

394. Mullin R. Cost to develop new pharmaceutical drug now exceeds $2.5 B. Scientific American. 2014;24.

395. Henry B. Drug Pricing & Challenges to Hepatitis C Treatment Access. J Health Biomed Law. 2018;14:265-83. Available from: https://pmc.ncbi.nlm.nih.gov/articles/PMC6152913/.

396. Mehdi Najafzadeh, Karin Andersson, William H. Shrank, Alexis A. Krumme, Olga S. Matlin, Troyen Brennan, et al. Cost-Effectiveness of Novel Regimens for the Treatment of Hepatitis C Virus. Annals of Internal Medicine. 2015;162(6):407-19. Available from: https://www.acpjournals.org/doi/abs/10.7326/M14-1152.

397. Prinz F, Schlange T, Asadullah K. Believe it or not: how much can we rely on published data on potential drug targets? Nat Rev Drug Discov. 2011;10(9):712-. Available from: http://dx.doi.org/10.1038/nrd3439-c1.

398. Ioannidis JPA. Why Most Clinical Research Is Not Useful. PLoS Med. 2016;13(6). Available from: https://journals.plos.org/plosmedicine/article?id=10.1371/journal.pmed.1002049.

399. Green RH. The association of viral activation with penicillin toxicity in guinea pigs and hamsters. The Yale journal of biology and medicine. 1974;47(3):166. Available from: https://pmc.ncbi.nlm.nih.gov/articles/PMC2595098/.

400. Alkhafaji AA, Trinquart L, Baron G, Desvarieux M, Ravaud P. Impact of evergreening on patients and health insurance: a meta analysis and reimbursement cost analysis of citalopram/escitalopram antidepressants. BMC Medicine. 2012;10(1):142. Available from: https://doi.org/10.1186/1741-7015-10-142.

401. Nguyen TM. Abuse-deterrent opioids: Worth the effort and cost? Chemical & Engineering News. 2018;95(45):34-6. Available from: https://cen.acs.org/articles/95/i45/Abuse-deterrent-opioids-Worth-effort.html.

402. Freeman DH. Lies, damned lies, and medical science. The Atlantic. 2010. Available from: http://www.theatlantic.com/magazine/archive/2010/11/lies-damned-lies-and-medical-science/308269/.

403. Horton R. Vioxx, the implosion of Merck, and aftershocks at the FDA. The Lancet. 2004;364(9450):1995-6. Available from: http://www.thelancet.com/journals/lancet/article/PIIS0140-6736(04)17523-5/abstract.

404. Krumholz HM, Ross JS, Presler AH, Egilman DS. What have we learnt from Vioxx? Bmj. 2007;334(7585):120-3. Available from: http://www.ncbi.nlm.nih.gov/pmc/articles/PMC1779871/pdf/bmj-334-7585-feat-00120.pdf.

405. SoRelle R. Withdrawal of Posicor from market. Circulation. 1998;98(9):831-2. Available from: http://circ.ahajournals.org/content/98/9/831.full.pdf.

406. Rockoff JD, Silverman E. Pharmaceutical Companies Buy Rivals' Drugs, Then Jack Up the Prices. Wall Street Journal. 2015 April 26, 2015. Available from: https://www.wsj.com/articles/pharmaceutical-companies-buy-rivals-drugs-then-jack-up-the-prices-1430096431.

407. Pollack A. Drug goes from $13.50 a tablet to $750, overnight. New York Times. 2015 September 20, 2015. Available from: https://www.nytimes.com/2015/09/21/business/a-huge-overnight-increase-in-a-drugs-price-raises-protests.html.

408. Rosenberg ME, Rosenberg SP. Changes in Retail Prices of Prescription Dermatologic Drugs From 2009 to 2015. JAMA dermatology. 2015:1-6. Available from: https://jamanetwork.com/journals/jamadermatology/fullarticle/2471623.

409. Crow D. Pfizer delays drug price rises after discussions with Trump. Financial Times. 2018 11/7/2018. Available from: https://www.ft.com/content/2e926b74-84aa-11e8-96dd-fa565ec55929.

410. Burns PB, Rohrich RJ, Chung KC. The levels of evidence and their role in evidence-based medicine. Plast Reconstr Surg. 2011;128(1):305-10. Available from: https://journals.lww.com/plasreconsurg/fulltext/2011/07000/the_levels_of_evidence_and_their_role_in.46.aspx

https://pmc.ncbi.nlm.nih.gov/articles/PMC3124652/pdf/nihms288127.pdf.

411. National Institute of Clinical Studies. Appendix F: Levels of evidence and recommendation grading. National Health and Medical Research Council,; 2009. Available from: https://www.nhmrc.gov.au/sites/default/files/images/appendix-f-levels-of-evidence.pdf.

412. Matheson A. Can self-regulation deliver an ethical commercial literature? A critical reading of the "Good Publication Practice" (GPP3) guidelines for industry-financed medical journal articles. Accountability in Research. 2019;26(2):85-107. Available from: https://doi.org/10.1080/08989621.2018.1564663.

413. Every-Palmer S, Howick J. How evidence-based medicine is failing due to biased trials and selective publication. Journal of Evaluation in Clinical Practice. 2014;20(6):908-14. Available from: https://onlinelibrary.wiley.com/doi/abs/10.1111/jep.12147.

414. Lim S, Hor C, Tay K, Mat Jelani A, Tan W, Ker H, et al. Efficacy of Ivermectin Treatment on Disease Progression Among Adults With Mild to Moderate COVID-19 and Comorbidities: The I-TECH Randomized Clinical Trial. JAMA Internal Medicine. 2022;182(4):426-35. Available from: https://doi.org/10.1001/jamainternmed.2022.0189.

415. Lewis JH, Kilgore ML, Goldman DP, Trimble EL, Kaplan R, Montello MJ, et al. Participation of patients 65 years of age or older in cancer clinical trials. J Clin Oncol. 2003;21(7):1383-9. Available from: https://ascopubs.org/doi/abs/10.1200/jco.2003.08.010

https://scholar.archive.org/work/ndrjsah5jzhs3ps6a5oxdjbuau/access/wayback/http://assets.wharton.upenn.edu:80/~housman/publications/jco.pdf.

416. Hutchins LF, Unger JM, Crowley JJ, Coltman CA, Albain KS. Underrepresentation of Patients 65 Years of Age or Older in Cancer-Treatment Trials. New England Journal of Medicine. 1999;341(27):2061-7. Available from: https://www.nejm.org/doi/full/10.1056/NEJM199912303412706.

417. Townsley CA, Selby R, Siu LL. Systematic Review of Barriers to the Recruitment of Older Patients With Cancer Onto Clinical Trials. Journal of Clinical Oncology. 2005;23(13):3112-24. Available from: https://ascopubs.org/doi/abs/10.1200/JCO.2005.00.141.

418. Sacher AG, Le LW, Leighl NB, Coate LE. Elderly Patients with Advanced NSCLC in Phase III Clinical Trials: Are the Elderly Excluded from Practice-Changing Trials in Advanced NSCLC? Journal of Thoracic Oncology. 2013;8(3):366-8. Available from: https://www.sciencedirect.com/science/article/pii/S1556086415327714.

419. Kemeny MM, Peterson BL, Kornblith AB, Muss HB, Wheeler J, Levine E, et al. Barriers to Clinical Trial Participation by Older Women With Breast Cancer. Journal of Clinical Oncology. 2003;21(12):2268-75. Available from: https://ascopubs.org/doi/abs/10.1200/JCO.2003.09.124.

420. Fitzsimmons PR, Blayney S, Mina-Corkill S, Scott GO. Older participants are frequently excluded from Parkinson's disease research. Parkinsonism & Related Disorders. 2012;18(5):585-9. Available from: https://www.sciencedirect.com/science/article/pii/S135380201200079X.

421. Reis G, Silva E, Silva D, Thabane L, Milagres A, Ferreira T, et al. Effect of Early Treatment with Ivermectin among Patients with Covid-19. New England Journal of Medicine. 2022;386(18):1721-31. Available from: https://www.nejm.org/doi/full/10.1056/NEJMoa2115869.

422. Marinos A. Do Your Own Research [Internet]: Substack. 2022. Available from: https://doyourownresearch.substack.com/p/the-problem-with-the-together-trial.

423. McGauran N, Wieseler B, Kreis J, Schüler Y-B, Kölsch H, Kaiser T. Reporting bias in medical research - a narrative review. Trials. 2010;11(1):37. Available from: https://doi.org/10.1186/1745-6215-11-37.

424. Lexchin J. Those Who Have the Gold Make the Evidence: How the Pharmaceutical Industry Biases the Outcomes of Clinical Trials of Medications. Science and Engineering Ethics. 2012;18(2):247-61. Available from: https://doi.org/10.1007/s11948-011-9265-3.

425. Matheson A. Marketing trials, marketing tricks — how to spot them and how to stop them. Trials. 2017;18(1):105. Available from: https://doi.org/10.1186/s13063-017-1827-5.

426. Probst P, Knebel P, Grummich K, Tenckhoff S, Ulrich A, Büchler M, et al. Industry Bias in Randomized Controlled Trials in General and Abdominal Surgery: An Empirical Study. Annals of Surgery. 2016;264(1):87-92. Available from: https://journals.lww.com/annalsofsurgery/fulltext/2016/07000/industry_bias_in_randomized_controlled_trials_in.15.aspx.

427. Hughes S, Cohen D, Jaggi R. Differences in reporting serious adverse events in industry sponsored clinical trial registries and journal articles on antidepressant and antipsychotic drugs: a cross-sectional study. BMJ Open. 2014;4(7):e005535. Available from: https://bmjopen.bmj.com/content/bmjopen/4/7/e005535.full.pdf.

428. Schroll JB, Penninga EI, Gøtzsche PC. Assessment of Adverse Events in Protocols, Clinical Study Reports, and Published Papers of Trials of Orlistat: A Document Analysis. PLoS Med. 2016;13(8):e1002101. Available from: https://doi.org/10.1371/journal.pmed.1002101.

429. Cherla D, Viso C, Holihan J, Bernardi K, Moses M, Mueck K, et al. The Effect of Financial Conflict of Interest, Disclosure Status, and Relevance on Medical Research from the United States. J Gen Intern Med. 2019;34(3):429-34. Available from: https://doi.org/10.1007/s11606-018-4784-0.

430. Harris R. Long-Term Studies Of COVID-19 Vaccines Hurt By Placebo Recipients Getting Immunized. NPR National Public Radio (US). 2021 February 19th, 2021. Available from: https://www.npr.org/sections/health-shots/2021/02/19/969143015/long-term-studies-of-covid-19-vaccines-hurt-by-placebo-recipients-getting-immuni.

431. Sismondo S. Pharmaceutical company funding and its consequences: A qualitative systematic review. Contemporary Clinical Trials. 2008;29(2):109-13. Available from: https://www.sciencedirect.com/science/article/pii/S1551714407001255.

432. Flacco M, Manzoli L, Boccia S, Capasso L, Aleksovska K, Rosso A, et al. Head-to-head randomized trials are mostly industry sponsored and almost always favor the industry sponsor. Journal of Clinical Epidemiology. 2015;68(7):811-20. Available from: https://www.sciencedirect.com/science/article/pii/S089543561500058X.

433. Bero L, Oostvogel F, Bacchetti P, Lee K. Factors Associated with Findings of Published Trials of Drug–Drug Comparisons: Why Some Statins Appear More Efficacious than Others. PLoS Med. 2007;4(6):e184. Available from: https://doi.org/10.1371/journal.pmed.0040184.

434. Light DW, Lexchin JR. Pharmaceuticals as a market for "lemons": Theory and practice. Social Science & Medicine. 2021;268:113368. Available from: https://www.sciencedirect.com/science/article/pii/S0277953620305876.

435. Light D, Lexchin J. Pharmaceuticals as a market for "lemons": Theory and practice. Social Science & Medicine. 2021;268:113368. Available from: https://www.sciencedirect.com/science/article/pii/S0277953620305876.

436. Doucet M, Sismondo S. Evaluating solutions to sponsorship bias. Journal of Medical Ethics. 2008;34(8):627-30. Available from: https://jme.bmj.com/content/medethics/34/8/627.full.pdf.

437. Ravnskov U, Alabdulgader A, de Lorgeril M, Diamond DM, Hama R, Hamazaki T, et al. The new European guidelines for prevention of cardiovascular disease are misleading. Expert review of clinical pharmacology. 2020;13(12):1289-94. Available from: https://www.tandfonline.com/doi/abs/10.1080/17512433.2020.1841635

https://www.researchgate.net/profile/Uffe-Ravnskov/publication/348359099_The_new_European_guidelines_for_prevention_of_cardiovascular_disease_are_misleading/links/6180f0ed3c987366c316fccb/The-new-European-guidelines-for-prevention-of-cardiovascular-disease-are-misleading.pdf.

438. Brown S. Most Dietary Guideline Advisors Have Ties to Food and Pharma Industries, Study Finds: Verywell Health; 2022 [Available from: https://www.verywellhealth.com/dietary-guidelines-committee-conflicts-of-interest-5223556.

439. Ioannidis JPA. Evidence-based medicine has been hijacked: a report to David Sackett. Journal of Clinical Epidemiology. 2016;73:82-6. Available from: http://www.sciencedirect.com/science/article/pii/S0895435616001475.

440. Chalmers I, Bracken MB, Djulbegovic B, Garattini S, Grant J, Gülmezoglu AM, et al. How to increase value and reduce waste when research priorities are set. The Lancet. 2014;383(9912):156-65. Available from: http://www.sciencedirect.com/science/article/pii/S0140673613622291.

441. Begley CG, Ioannidis JPA. Reproducibility in Science: Improving the Standard for Basic and Preclinical Research. Circulation Research. 2015;116(1):116-26. Available from: http://circres.ahajournals.org/content/116/1/116.abstract.

442. Ioannidis JP. How to make more published research true. PLoS Med. 2014;11(10):e1001747. Available from: https://www.ncbi.nlm.nih.gov/pubmed/25334033.

443. Ioannidis JPA, Greenland S, Hlatky MA, Khoury MJ, Macleod MR, Moher D, et al. Increasing value and reducing waste in research design, conduct, and analysis. The Lancet. 2014;383(9912):166-75. Available from: http://www.sciencedirect.com/science/article/pii/S0140673613622278.

444. Begley CG, Ellis LM. Drug development: Raise standards for preclinical cancer research. Nature. 2012;483(7391):531-3. Available from: http://www.ncbi.nlm.nih.gov/pubmed/22460880.

445. Hanson JD, Kysar DA. Taking Behavioralism Seriously: Some Evidence of Market Manipulation. Harvard Law Review. 1999;112(7):1420-572. Available from: http://www.jstor.org/stable/1342413.

446. Trinquart L, Johns DM, Galea S. Why do we think we know what we know? A metaknowledge analysis of the salt controversy. International Journal of Epidemiology. 2016. Available from: http://ije.oxfordjournals.org/content/early/2016/02/17/ije.dyv184.abstract.

447. Cobb LK, Anderson CA, Elliott P, Hu FB, Liu K, Neaton JD, et al. Methodological Issues in Cohort Studies That Relate Sodium Intake to Cardiovascular Disease Outcomes A Science Advisory From the American Heart Association. Circulation. 2014;129(10):1173-86. Available from: https://www.ahajournals.org/doi/full/10.1161/CIR.0000000000000015

https://www.ahajournals.org/doi/pdf/10.1161/CIR.0000000000000015.

448. Ravnskov U. The benefits of high cholesterol. Well Being Journal. 2004;43. Available from: http://www.reboundhealth.com/cms/images/pdf/Article-by-Various-Authors/benefits%20of%20high%20cholesterol%20by%20uffe%20ravnskov%20md%20phd%20id%2019128.pdf.

449. Ravnskov U. Cholesterol was healthy in the end. A Balanced Omega-6/Omega-3 Fatty Acid Ratio, Cholesterol and Coronary Heart Disease. 2009;100:90-109. Available from: https://karger.com/books/book/2670/chapter-abstract/5753173/Cholesterol-Was-Healthy-in-the-End

https://scholar.archive.org/work/mnuo3lged5e3zbmyyccmfzdg4a/access/wayback/http://pdfs.semanticscholar.org/ab76/d7d9cccac85c9746e489f5a75820bbee29e5.pdf.

450. Ravnskov U, DiNicolantonio JJ, Harcombe Z, Kummerow FA, Okuyama H, Worm N, editors. The questionable benefits of exchanging saturated fat with polyunsaturated fat. Mayo Clinic Proceedings; 2014: Elsevier. Available from: https://www.mayoclinicproceedings.org/article/S0025-6196(13)01004-5/fulltext

https://www.mayoclinicproceedings.org/article/S0025-6196(13)01004-5/pdf.

451. Okuyama H. 6. Benefits of high cholesterol levels for all-cause mortality: biochemical bases. In: Watson R, Meester FD, editors. Handbook of eggs in human function: Wageningen Academic Publihers; 2015. p. 93-108. Available from: https://www.wageningenacademic.com/doi/abs/10.3920/978-90-8686-804-9_6.

452. Ellison LF, Morrison HI. Low Serum Cholesterol Concentration and Risk of Suicide. Epidemiology. 2001;12(2):168-72. Available from: https://journals.lww.com/epidem/fulltext/2001/03000/low_serum_cholesterol_concentration_and_risk_of.7.aspx.

453. Page IH, Allen EV, Chamberlain FL, Keys A, Stamler J, Stare FJ. Dietary fat and its relation to heart attacks and strokes.

Report by the Central Committee for Medical and Community Program of the American Heart Association. JAMA. 1961;175:389-91. Available from: https://www.ahajournals.org/doi/abs/10.1161/01.cir.23.1.133

https://www.ahajournals.org/doi/pdf/10.1161/01.cir.23.1.133.

454. Ravnskov U, Diamond DM, Hama R, Hamazaki T, Hammarskjöld B, Hynes N, et al. Lack of an association or an inverse association between low-density-lipoprotein cholesterol and mortality in the elderly: a systematic review. BMJ open. 2016;6(6):e010401. Available from: https://bmjopen.bmj.com/content/6/6/e010401?fbclid=IwAR2ctrIBpjoUjAZcdtdMhAt3U4b_J-9TYSEIXda51TCRGYNqrO12GRABXvM.

455. Economist TCH. What is "healthy"? The Economist. 2016 16/5/2016. Available from: http://www.economist.com/node/21698823/print; http://www.economist.com/blogs/economist-explains/2016/05/economist-explains-12.

456. Means C, Means C. Good Energy

The Surprising Connection Between Metabolism and Limitless Health. New York: Avery Penguin Random House; 2024.

457. Economist T. Tsinghua University may soon top the world league in science research. The Economist. 2018. Available from: https://www.economist.com/china/2018/11/17/tsinghua-university-may-soon-top-the-world-league-in-science-research.

458. Shariff SZ, Bejaimal SAD, Sontrop JM, Iansavichus AV, Haynes RB, Weir MA, et al. Retrieving Clinical Evidence: A Comparison of PubMed and Google Scholar for Quick Clinical Searches. Journal of Medical Internet Research. 2013;15(8):e164. Available from: http://www.ncbi.nlm.nih.gov/pmc/articles/PMC3757915/.

459. Shaw CA. Weaponizing the Peer Review System. International Journal of Vaccine Theory, Practice, and Research. 2020;1(1):11-26. Available from: https://doi.org/10.56098/ijvtpr.v1i1.1.

460. Smith R. Peer review: a flawed process at the heart of science and journals. Journal of the Royal Society of Medicine. 2006;99(4):178-82. Available from: http://www.ncbi.nlm.nih.gov/pmc/articles/PMC1420798/.

461. Smith R. Classical peer review: an empty gun. Breast Cancer Res. 2010;12(Suppl 4):S13. Available from: https://link.springer.com/article/10.1186/bcr2742.

462. MacDonald F. 8 scientific papers that were rejected before going on to win a Nobel prize. Science Alert, August. 2016;19. Available from: https://www.sciencealert.com/these-8-papers-were-rejected-before-going-on-to-win-the-nobel-prize.

463. Van Noorden R. Open Access: The true cost of science publishing. Nature. 2013;495(7442):426-9. Available from: https://www.nature.com/articles/495426a

https://rubiola.org/pdf-lectures/Scient-Public-Files/vanNoorden-2013.pdf.

464. Craig ID, Plume AM, McVeigh ME, Pringle J, Amin M. Do open access articles have greater citation impact?: A critical review of the literature. Journal of Informetrics. 2007;1(3):239-48. Available from: https://www.sciencedirect.com/science/article/pii/S1751157707000466.

465. Beall J. Beall's List of Predatory Publishers 2016 2016 [Available from: https://beallslist.net/.

466. Brundy C, Thornton JB. The paper mill crisis is a five-alarm fire for science: what can librarians do about it? Insights: the UKSG journal. 2024. Available from: https://insights.uksg.org/articles/10.1629/uksg.659.

467. Jefferson T, Alderson P, Wager E, Davidoff F. Effects of editorial peer review: A systematic review. JAMA. 2002;287(21):2784-6. Available from: http://dx.doi.org/10.1001/jama.287.21.2784.

468. Collective C. Ivermectin for COVID-19 in adults in the community (PRINCIPLE): an open, randomised, controlled, adaptive platform trial of short- and longer-term outcomes 2024 [updated February 2024. Available from: https://c19ivm.org/principleivm.html.

469. Specter M. The power of nothing. The New Yorker. 2011;87:12. Available from: http://www.newyorker.com/magazine/2011/12/12/the-power-of-nothing.

470. Chan A-W, Song F, Vickers A, Jefferson T, Dickersin K, Gøtzsche PC, et al. Increasing value and reducing waste: addressing inaccessible research. The Lancet. 2014;383(9913):257-66. Available from: http://www.sciencedirect.com/science/article/pii/S0140673613622965.

471. Glasziou P, Altman DG, Bossuyt P, Boutron I, Clarke M, Julious S, et al. Reducing waste from incomplete or unusable reports of biomedical research. The Lancet. 2014;383(9913):267-76. Available from: http://www.sciencedirect.com/science/article/pii/S014067361362228X.

472. Macleod MR, Michie S, Roberts I, Dirnagl U, Chalmers I, Ioannidis JP, et al. Biomedical research: increasing value, reducing waste. The Lancet.

2014;383(9912):101-4. Available from: http://www.thelancet.com/journals/lancet/article/PIIS0140-6736(13)62329-6/abstract.

473. Salman RA-S, Beller E, Kagan J, Hemminki E, Phillips RS, Savulescu J, et al. Increasing value and reducing waste in biomedical research regulation and management. The Lancet. 2014;383(9912):176-85. Available from: http://www.sciencedirect.com/science/article/pii/S0140673613622977.

474. Pocock SJ, Elbourne DR. Randomized trials or observational tribulations? New England Journal of Medicine. 2000;342(25):1907-9. Available from: https://www.nejm.org/doi/full/10.1056/NEJM200006223422511?url_ver=Z39.88-2003&rfr_id=ori%3Arid%3Acrossref.org&rfr_dat=cr_pub%3Dpubmed.

475. Concato J, Shah N, Horwitz RI. Randomized, Controlled Trials, Observational Studies, and the Hierarchy of Research Designs. New England Journal of Medicine. 2000;342(25):1887-92. Available from: https://www.nejm.org/doi/full/10.1056/NEJM200006223422507.

476. Benson K, Hartz AJ. A Comparison of Observational Studies and Randomized, Controlled Trials. New England Journal of Medicine. 2000;342(25):1878-86. Available from: https://www.nejm.org/doi/full/10.1056/NEJM200006223422506.

477. Silverman SL. From Randomized Controlled Trials to Observational Studies. The American Journal of Medicine. 2009;122(2):114-20. Available from: https://www.sciencedirect.com/science/article/pii/S0002934308009522.

478. Kunz R. Randomized trials and observational studies: still mostly similar results, still crucial differences. Journal of Clinical Epidemiology. 2008;61(3):207-8. Available from: https://doi.org/10.1016/j.jclinepi.2007.05.021.

479. Soni PD, Hartman HE, Dess RT, Abugharib A, Allen SG, Feng FY, et al. Comparison of Population-Based Observational Studies With Randomized Trials in Oncology. Journal of Clinical Oncology. 2019;37(14):1209-16. Available from: https://ascopubs.org/doi/abs/10.1200/JCO.18.01074.

480. Bosdriesz JR, Stel VS, van Diepen M, Meuleman Y, Dekker FW, Zoccali C, et al. Evidence-based medicine—When observational studies are better than randomized controlled trials. Nephrology. 2020;25(10):737-43. Available from: https://onlinelibrary.wiley.com/doi/abs/10.1111/nep.13742.

481. Coleman K, Norris S, Weston A, Grimmer-Somers K, Hillier S, Merlin T, et al. NHMRC additional levels of evidence and grades for recommendations for developers of guidelines. Canberra: NHMRC. 2009. Available from: https://www.mja.com.au/sites/default/files/NHMRC.levels.of.evidence.2008-09.pdf.

482. Simpson JA, Weiner ES. The Oxford english dictionary: Clarendon Press Oxford; 1989.

483. Palmer CR. Encyclopedia of Biostatistics. BMJ. 1999;318(7182):542. Available from: http://www.bmj.com/content/bmj/318/7182/542.1.full.pdf.

484. Guyatt G, Cairns J, Churchill D, Cook D, Haynes B, Hirsh J, et al. Evidence-Based Medicine: A New Approach to Teaching the Practice of Medicine.

JAMA. 1992;268(17):2420-5. Available from: https://doi.org/10.1001/jama.1992.03490170092032.

485. Sackett D, Ellis J, Mulligan I, Rowe J. Inpatient general medicine is evidence based. The Lancet. 1995;346(8972):407-10. Available from: https://www.thelancet.com/journals/lancet/article/PIIS0140-6736(95)92781-6/fulltext

https://www.thelancet.com/pdfs/journals/lancet/PIIS0140-6736(95)92781-6.pdf.

486. Geddes J, Game D, Jenkins N, Peterson L, Pottinger G, Sackett D, editors. In-patient psychiatric care is evidence-based. Proceedings of the Royal College of Psychiatrists Winter Meeting, Stratford/UK; 1996.

487. Committee for Evaluating Medical Technologies in Clinical Use, Eddy D. Assessing Medical Technologies. p.5 National Academy of Sciences, Division of Health Sciences Policy, Division of Health Promotion and Disease Prevention; 1985. Available from: http://www.nap.edu/catalog/607.html.

488. Greenhalgh T. "Is my practice evidence-based?". BMJ. 1996;313(7063):957. Available from: http://www.bmj.com/content/313/7063/957.abstract.

489. Angell M. The truth about the drug companies: How they deceive us and what to do about it: Random House Trade Paperbacks New York; 2005.

490. Akerlof GA, Shiller RJ. Phishing for phools: The economics of manipulation and deception: Princeton University Press; 2015.

491. Demasi M. Cochrane–a sinking ship? BMJ EBM Spotlight blog. 2018;16. Available from: https://blogs.bmj.com/bmjebmspotlight/2018/09/16/cochrane-a-sinking-ship/

492. Gøtzsche PC. The decline and fall of the Cochrane empire. 2022. Available from: https://www.scientificfreedom.dk/wp-content/uploads/2022/01/Gotzsche-Decline-and-fall-of-the-Cochrane-empire.pdf.

493. Nass M, Noble Jr JH. Whither Cochrane. Indian J Med Ethics Epub. 2018. Available from: https://www.researchgate.net/profile/John-Noble-Jr/publication/349870446_Unraveling_the_medical-industrial_complex_confessions_of_a_reformed_sinner/links/6071b00aa6fdcc5f77969d9b/Unraveling-the-medical-industrial-complex-confessions-of-a-reformed-sinner.pdf.

494. Ahmad AS, Ormiston-Smith N, Sasieni PD. Trends in the lifetime risk of developing cancer in Great Britain: comparison of risk for those born from 1930 to 1960. Br J Cancer. 2015;112(5):943-7. Available from: http://dx.doi.org/10.1038/bjc.2014.606.

495. CDC Centers for Disease Control and Prevention. Trends in Current Cigarette Smoking Among High School Students and Adults, United States, 1965–2014 2016 [Available from: http://www.cdc.gov/tobacco/data_statistics/tables/trends/cig_smoking/.

496. Schmutz A, Matta M, Cairat M, Espina C, Schüz J, Kampman E, et al. Mapping the European cancer prevention research landscape: A case for more prevention research funding. European Journal of Cancer. 2023;195:113378. Available from: https://www.sciencedirect.com/science/article/pii/S0959804923006809.

497. Meyskens FL, Jr, Mukhtar H, Rock CL, Cuzick J, Kensler TW, Yang CS, et al. Cancer Prevention: Obstacles, Challenges, and the Road Ahead. JNCI: Journal of the National Cancer Institute. 2015;108(2). Available from: https://doi.org/10.1093/jnci/djv309.

498. Carter AJR, Nguyen CN. A comparison of cancer burden and research spending reveals discrepancies in the distribution of research funding. BMC Public Health. 2012;12(1):526. Available from: https://doi.org/10.1186/1471-2458-12-526.

499. Silberzahn R. UEL, Martin D. P., Anselmi P., Aust F., Awtrey E., Bahník Š., Bai F., Bannard C., Bonnier E., Carlsson R., Cheung F., Christensen G., Clay R., , Craig M. A. DRA, Dam L., Evans M. H., Flores Cervantes I., Fong N., Gamez-Djokic M., Glenz A., Gordon-McKeon S., Heaton T. J., Hederos Eriksson K., Heene M., Hofelich Mohr A. J., Högden F., Hui K., Johannesson M., Kalodimos J., Kaszubowski E., Kennedy D.M., Lei R., Lindsay T. A., Liverani S., Madan C. R., Molden D., Molleman E., Morey R. D., Mulder L. B., Nijstad B. R., Pope N. G., Pope B., Prenoveau J. M., Rink F., Robusto E., Roderique H., Sandberg A., Schlüter E., Schönbrodt F. D., Sherman M. F., Sommer S.A., Sotak K., Spain S., Spörlein C., Stafford T., Stefanutti L., Tauber S., Ullrich J., Vianello M., Wagenmakers E.J., Witkowiak M., Yoon S., Nosek B. A. Many analysts, one dataset: Making transparent how variations in analytical choices affect results. Open Science Framework. 2016. Available from: https://osf.io/j5v8f/.

500. Aschwanden C. Failure Is Moving Science Forward FiveThirtyEight. 2016. Available from: http://fivethirtyeight.com/features/failure-is-moving-science-forward/.

501. Aschwanden C, King R. Science isn't broken, FiveThirtyEight. 2015. Available from: https://fivethirtyeight.com/features/science-isnt-broken/.

502. Coase RH. Essays on economics and economists: University of Chicago Press; 1995.

503. World Medical Association. World Medical Association Declaration of Helsinki. Ethical principles for medical research involving human subjects. Bulletin of the World Health Organization. 2001;79(4):373. Available from: https://pmc.ncbi.nlm.nih.gov/articles/PMC2566407/

https://pmc.ncbi.nlm.nih.gov/articles/PMC2566407/pdf/11357217.pdf.

504. Cypreste R, Walsh K, Bedford M. Evidence-based medicine: what does the future hold? Postgraduate Medical Journal. 2015;91(1077):359-60. Available from: http://pmj.bmj.com/content/91/1077/359.short.

505. Fortin M, Dionne J, Pinho G, Gignac J, Almirall J, Lapointe L. Randomized Controlled Trials: Do They Have External Validity for Patients With Multiple Comorbidities? The Annals of Family Medicine. 2006;4(2):104-8. Available from: http://www.annfammed.org/content/4/2/104.abstract.

506. Pirmohamed M, James S, Meakin S, Green C, Scott AK, Walley TJ, et al. Adverse drug reactions as cause of admission to hospital: prospective analysis of 18 820 patients. BMJ. 2004;329(7456):15. Available from: http://www.bmj.com/content/329/7456/15.abstract.

507. Parnell S. Natural therapy cover risk to private health rebate. The Australian. 2015. Available from: http://www.theaustralian.com.au/national-affairs/health/natural-therapy-cover-risk-to-private-health-rebate/news-story/aa9a1f5c69048d1ba538fa8ed8149636.

508. Molassiotis A, Fernadez-Ortega P, Pud D, Ozden G, Scott JA, Panteli V, et al. Use of complementary and alternative medicine in cancer patients: a European survey. Annals of oncology. 2005;16(4):655-63. Available from: http://annonc.oxfordjournals.org/content/16/4/655.full.pdf.

509. Nahin RL, Barnes PM, Stussman BJ, Bloom B. Costs of complementary and alternative medicine (CAM) and frequency of visits to CAM practitioners: United States, 2007. Natl Health Stat Report. 2009;18(18):1-14. Available from: https://stacks.cdc.gov/view/cdc/11548

https://stacks.cdc.gov/view/cdc/11548/cdc_11548_DS1.pdf.

510. Bodeker G, Kronenberg F. A Public Health Agenda for Traditional, Complementary, and Alternative Medicine. American Journal of Public Health. 2002;92(10):1582-91. Available from: http://dx.doi.org/10.2105/AJPH.92.10.1582.

511. Goldbeck-Wood S, Dorozynski A, Lie LG, Yamauchi M, Zinn C, Josefson D, et al. Complementary medicine is booming worldwide. Br Med J. 1996;313(7050):131-4. Available from: https://www.bmj.com/content/313/7050/131.1.

512. Pagán JA, Pauly MV. Access To Conventional Medical Care And The Use Of Complementary And Alternative Medicine. Health Affairs. 2005;24(1):255-62. Available from: http://content.healthaffairs.org/content/24/1/255.abstract.

513. Ioannidis JP. Why most discovered true associations are inflated. Epidemiology. 2008;19(5):640-8. Available from: https://journals.lww.com/epidem/fulltext/2008/09000/The_Emergence_of_Networks_in_Human_Genome.2.aspx.

514. Cumming G. Understanding the new statistics: Effect sizes, confidence intervals, and meta-analysis: Routledge; 2013.

515. Cumming G. Intro Statistics 9 Dance of the p Values. 2013. Available from: https://www.youtube.com/watch?v=5OL1RqHrZQ8.

516. Smith G. Standard Deviations: Flawed Assumptions, Tortured Data, and Other Ways to Lie with Statistics: Penguin; 2014.

517. Huff D. How to lie with statistics (illust. I. Geis). NY: Norton. 1954.

518. Huff D. How to lie with statistics: WW Norton & Company; 1993.

519. Webb P, Bain C. Essential epidemiology: an introduction for students and health professionals: Cambridge University Press; 2010.

520. Kannel WB, McGee DL. Diabetes and cardiovascular disease: the Framingham study. Jama. 1979;241(19):2035-8. Available from: https://jamanetwork.com/journals/jama/article-abstract/364764.

521. GRADE Working Group. Grading quality of evidence and strength of recommendations. BMJ : British Medical Journal. 2004;328(7454):1490-.

Available from: http://www.ncbi.nlm.nih.gov/pmc/articles/ PMC428525/.

522. NHMRC. How to use the evidence: assessment and application of scientific evidence. In: Council NHaMR, editor. Web: Australian Government; 2000. Available from: https://www.nhmrc.gov.au/_files_nhmrc/publications/ attachments/cp69.pdf.

523. Kamangar F, Qiao YL, Blaser MJ, Sun XD, Katki H, Fan JH, et al. Helicobacter pylori and oesophageal and gastric cancers in a prospective study in China. British Journal of Cancer. 2007;96(1):172-6. Available from: https:// doi.org/10.1038/sj.bjc.6603517.

524. Webb PM, Yu MC, Forman D, Henderson BE, Newell DG, Yuan J-M, et al. An apparent lack of association between Helicobacter pylori infection and risk of gastric cancer in China. International Journal of Cancer. 1996;67(5):603-7. Available from: https://onlinelibrary.wiley.com/doi/ abs/10.1002/%28SICI%291097-0215%2819960904%2967%3A5%3C603% 3A%3AAID-IJC2%3E3.0.CO%3B2-Y.

525. Hariton E, Locascio JJ. Randomised controlled trials – the gold standard for effectiveness research. BJOG: An International Journal of Obstetrics & Gynaecology. 2018;125(13):1716-. Available from: https://obgyn. onlinelibrary.wiley.com/doi/abs/10.1111/1471-0528.15199.

526. Meldrum ML. A Brief History of the Randomized Controlled Trial:: From Oranges and Lemons to the Gold Standard. Hematology/Oncology Clinics of North America. 2000;14(4):745-60. Available from: https://www. sciencedirect.com/science/article/pii/S0889858805703099.

527. Vardakas KZ, Siempos II, Grammatikos A, Athanassa Z, Korbila IP, Falagas ME. Respiratory fluoroquinolones for the treatment of community-acquired pneumonia: a meta-analysis of randomized controlled trials. Canadian Medical Association Journal. 2008;179(12):1269-77. Available from: https://www.cmaj.ca/content/179/12/1269.short

https://www.cmaj.ca/content/cmaj/179/12/1269.full.pdf.

528. Myung S-K, Ju W, Cho B, Oh S-W, Park SM, Koo B-K, et al. Efficacy of vitamin and antioxidant supplements in prevention of cardiovascular disease: systematic review and meta-analysis of randomised controlled trials. BMJ. 2013;346. Available from: http://www.bmj.com/bmj/346/bmj.f10. full.pdf.

529. King M, Nazareth I, Lampe F, et al. Impact of participant and physician intervention preferences on randomized trials: A systematic review. JAMA. 2005;293(9):1089-99. Available from: http://dx.doi.org/10.1001/ jama.293.9.1089.

530. Kory P. Pierre Kory's Medical Musings [Internet]: Substack. 2024. [cited 2024]. Available from: https://pierrekorymedicalmusings.com/p/ the-last-of-the-big-seven-fraudulent.

531. Kory P. The Digger [Internet]: Substack. 2024. [cited 2024]. Available from: https://philharper.substack.com/p/ivermectin-and-the-research-cartel.

532. Ioannidis JPA. The Mass Production of Redundant, Misleading, and Conflicted Systematic Reviews and Meta-analyses. The Milbank Quarterly. 2016;94(3):485-514. Available from: http://dx.doi.org/10.1111/1468-0009.12210.

533. Munroe R. P-Values: xkcd.com; 2015 [Available from: https://xkcd.com/1478 http://imgs.xkcd.com/comics/p_values.png

534. Allison DB, Brown AW, George BJ, Kaiser KA. Reproducibility: A tragedy of errors. Nature. 2016;530(7588):27-9. Available from: https://www.nature.com/articles/530027a https://www.nature.com/articles/530027a.pdf.

535. Marcus A, Oransky I. Retraction Watch Tracking retractions as a window into the scientific progress 2024 [Available from: https://retractionwatch.com/.

536. Elisha E, Guetzkow J, Shir-Raz Y, Ronel N. Retraction of scientific papers: the case of vaccine research. Critical Public Health. 2022;32(4):533-42. Available from: https://doi.org/10.1080/09581596.2021.1878109.

537. Simonsohn U, Nelson L, Simmons J. Data Colada [Internet]2024. [cited 2024]. Available from: https://datacolada.org/.

538. Rekdal OB. Academic urban legends. Social Studies of Science. 2014;44(4):638-54. Available from: https://journals.sagepub.com/doi/full/10.1177/0306312714535679.

539. Dubner SJ. Why Is There So Such Fraud in Academia [Internet]: Stitcher and Renbud Radio; 2024. Podcast: 79:43. Available from: https://freakonomics.com/podcast/why-is-there-so-much-fraud-in-academia/

540. Karcz M, Papadakos PJ. The Consequences of Fraud and Deceit in Medical Research. Canadian Journal of Respiratory Therapy. 2011;47(1):18-27. Available from: https://www.proquest.com/openview/d9161a7ad2b286 00dab4bbef1616f5f6/1?pq-origsite=gscholar&cbl=32646.

541. Kaplan RM, Irvin VL. Likelihood of null effects of large NHLBI clinical trials has increased over time XX. PloS one. 2015;10(8):e0132382. Available from: http://www.ncbi.nlm.nih.gov/pmc/articles/PMC4526697/pdf/pone.0132382.pdf.

542. Woolston C. Registered clinical trials make positive findings vanish ZZZ. nature. 2015;524(7565). Available from: http://www.nature.com/news/registered-clinical-trials-make-positive-findings-vanish-1.18181.

543. Australian Bureau of Statistics. Overweight and Obesity. 2013. Available from: http://www.abs.gov.au/ausstats/abs@.nsf/Lookup/by%20 Subject/4338.0~2011-13~Main%20Features~Overweight%20and%20 obesity~10007.

544. Champkin J. "We need the public to become better BS detectors": Sir Iain Chalmers. Significance. 2014;11(3):25-30. Available from: https://academic.oup.com/jrssig/article-abstract/11/3/25/7029010 https://rss.onlinelibrary.wiley.com/doi/pdfdirect/10.1111/j.1740-9713.2014.00751.x.

545. Staff N. NHMRC Research Funding Facts Book 2013. NHMRC; 2013. Available from: https://www.nhmrc.gov.au/_files_nhmrc/publications/attachments/nh167_funding_facts_book_2013.pdf.

546. Barnett AG, Graves N, Clarke P, Herbert D. The impact of a streamlined funding application process on application time: two cross-sectional surveys of Australian researchers. BMJ open. 2015;5(1):e006912. Available from: http://www.ncbi.nlm.nih.gov/pmc/articles/PMC4298094/pdf/bmjopen-2014-006912.pdf.

547. clinicaltrials.gov. FDAAA 801 Requirements for clinical trial registrations. In: Health NIo, editor. 2016. Available from: https://clinicaltrials.gov/ct2/manage-recs/fdaaa

https://www.gpo.gov/fdsys/pkg/PLAW-110publ85/html/PLAW-110publ85.htm.

548. Smaldino PE, McElreath R. The natural selection of bad science. Royal Society Open Science. 2016;3(9). Available from: https://royalsocietypublishing.org/doi/full/10.1098/rsos.160384.

549. PLOS One Search. Ioannidis 2005 Paper Most Downloaded Paper of all time, 4x second placed paper 2016 [Available from: http://journals.plos.org/plosmedicine/search?unformattedQuery=%28publication_date%3A%5B2000-01-01T00%3A00%3A00Z+TO+2016-03-31T00%3A00%3A00Z%5D%29+AND+subject%3A%22%2FBiology+and+life+sciences%22&sortOrder=MOST_VIEWS_ALL_TIME.

550. Chakma J, Sun GH, Steinberg JD, Sammut SM, Jagsi R. Asia's ascent—global trends in biomedical R&D expenditures. New England Journal of Medicine. 2014;370(1):3-6. Available from: https://www.nejm.org/doi/abs/10.1056/NEJMp1311068.

551. NCSES National Center for Science and Engineering Statistics. U.S. and Global Research and Development

Up to 2019: NCSES National Center for Science and Engineering Statistics; 2022 [Available from: https://ncses.nsf.gov/pubs/nsb20221/u-s-and-global-research-and-development.

552. Moses HI, Matheson DM, Cairns-Smith S, George BP, Palisch C, Dorsey E. The anatomy of medical research: US and international comparisons. JAMA. 2015;313(2):174-89. Available from: http://dx.doi.org/10.1001/jama.2014.15939.

553. Van Noorden R. Nature. 2014. [cited 2016]. Available from: http://blogs.nature.com/news/2014/05/global-scientific-output-doubles-every-nine-years.html.

554. Benhayon S. The Way of Initiation 2008.

555. Ekelund RB, Hébert RF, Tollison RD. An economic model of the medieval church: usury as a form of rent seeking. Journal of law, economics, & organization. 1989;5(2):307-31. Available from: https://academic.oup.com/jleo/article-abstract/5/2/307/801885

https://web.stanford.edu/~avner/Greif_228_2005/Ekelund%20et%20al%201989%20Usury%20JLEO.pdf.

556. Morris C. The Papal Monarchy: The Western Church from 1050 to 1250: The Western Church from 1050 to 1250: Clarendon Press; 1989.

557. Carlin M, Rosenthal JT. Food and eating in medieval Europe: Bloomsbury Publishing; 1998.

558. Dyer C. An age of transition. Economy and society in England in the later Middle Ages. 2005:24-5,130.

559. Friends of Science in Medicine. Summary of Principles 2016 [Available from: http://www.scienceinmedicine.org.au/index.php?option=com_content&view=article&id=177&Itemid=153.

560. Phelps K. Evidence aplenty for complementary medicines The Australian. 2012. Available from: http://www.theaustralian.com.au/news/health-science/evidence-aplenty-for-complementary-medicines/story-e6frg8y6-1226495660429.

561. Vagg M. Medicandus [Internet]: The Conversation. 2012. [cited 2016]. Available from: https://theconversation.com/why-science-in-medicine-needs-all-the-friends-it-can-get-6053.

562. Marron L. Friends of science in medicine: "Integrative medicine" has no place in universities. Australasian Science. 2015;36(6):46. Available from: https://search.informit.org/doi/10.3316/ielapa.536894564249506.

563. Moynihan R. Assaulting alternative medicine: worthwhile or witch hunt? BMJ. 2012;344. Available from: http://www.bmj.com/content/bmj/344/bmj.e1075.full.pdf.

564. Jones JM. In U.S., 3 in 10 Say They Take the Bible Literally: Gallup; 2011 [Available from: http://www.gallup.com/poll/148427/say-bible-literally.aspx.

565. Colquhoun D. 2009. [cited 2016]. Available from: http://www.dcscience.net/2009/01/15/most-alternative-medicine-is-illegal/.

566. Goldacre B. Bad science: quacks, hacks, and big pharma flacks: McClelland & Stewart; 2010.

567. Cutler DM, Rosen AB, Vijan S. The Value of Medical Spending in the United States, 1960–2000. New England Journal of Medicine. 2006;355(9):920-7. Available from: http://www.nejm.org/doi/full/10.1056/NEJMsa054744.

568. Sumner P, Vivian-Griffiths S, Boivin J, Williams A, Venetis CA, Davies A, et al. The association between exaggeration in health related science news and academic press releases: retrospective observational study. Bmj. 2014;349:g7015. Available from: https://www.bmj.com/content/349/bmj.G7015.abstract.

569. Stryker JE. Reporting Medical Information: Effects of Press Releases and Newsworthiness on Medical Journal Articles' Visibility in the News Media. Preventive Medicine. 2002;35(5):519-30. Available from: http://www.sciencedirect.com/science/article/pii/S0091743502911023.

570. Woloshin S, Schwartz LM, Casella SL, Kennedy AT, Larson RJ. Press Releases by Academic Medical Centers: Not So Academic? Annals of Internal Medicine. 2009;150(9):613-8. Available from: http://dx.doi. org/10.7326/0003-4819-150-9-200905050-00007.

571. Yavchitz A, Boutron I, Bafeta A, Marroun I, Charles P, Mantz J, et al. Misrepresentation of randomized controlled trials in press releases and news coverage: a cohort study. PLoS Med. 2012;9(9):e1001308. Available from: https://journals.plos.org/plosmedicine/article?id=10.1371/journal. pmed.1001308.

572. Ng M, Fleming T, Robinson M, Thomson B, Graetz N, Margono C, et al. Global, regional, and national prevalence of overweight and obesity in children and adults during 1980–2013: a systematic analysis for the Global Burden of Disease Study 2013. The Lancet. 2014;384(9945):766-81. Available from: https://www. thelancet.com/journals/lancet/article/PIIS0140-6736(14)60460-8/abstract ?jobId=1138&record=14&sort=4&category=1

https://www.ncbi.nlm.nih.gov/pmc/articles/PMC4624264/.

573. Blaser MJ. Missing Microbes: How the Overuse of Antibiotics is Fueling our Modern Plagues2014.

574. Mozumdar A, Liguori G. Persistent increase of prevalence of metabolic syndrome among US adults: NHANES III to NHANES 1999–2006. Diabetes care. 2011;34(1):216-9. Available from: https://diabetesjournals.org/care/ article/34/1/216/27470/Persistent-Increase-of-Prevalence-of-Metabolic.

575. Kelly MP, Capewell S. Relative contributions of changes in risk factors and treatment to the reduction in coronary heart disease mortality. Health Development Agency Briefing Paper. 2004. Available from: https:// citeseerx.ist.psu.edu/document?repid=rep1&type=pdf&doi=76d7e7eeea 5094939877f5fc4c5460bd0e231def.

576. Tunstall-Pedoe H, Kuulasmaa K, Mähönen M, Tolonen H, Ruokokoski E, Amouyel P. Contribution of trends in survival and coronar y-event rates to changes in coronary heart disease mortality: 10-year results from 37 WHO MONICA Project populations. Lancet. 1999;353(9164):1547-57. Available from: https://www.thelancet.com/journals/lancet/article/ PIIS0140-6736(99)04021-0/abstract.

577. Steinberg E, Greenfield S, Wolman DM, Mancher M, Graham R. Clinical practice guidelines we can trust: national academies press; 2011.

578. Jena AB, Prasad V, Goldman DP, Romley J. Mortality and treatment patterns among patients hospitalized with acute cardiovascular conditions during dates of national cardiology meetings. JAMA Internal Medicine. 2015;175(2):237-44. Available from: http://dx.doi.org/10.1001/jamainternmed.2014.6781.

579. Begley CG. Reproducibility: Six red flags for suspect work. Nature. 2013;497(7450):433-4. Available from: http://dx.doi.org/10.1038/497433a

http://www.ncbi.nlm.nih.gov/pubmed/23698428.

580. Yong E. Replication studies: Bad copy

In the wake of high profile controversies, psychologists are facing up to problems with replication. Nature. 2012;483:298-300. Available from: https://openurl.ebsco.com/EPDB%3Agcd%3A2%3A6289314/detailv2?si d=ebsco%3Aplink%3Ascholar&id=ebsco%3Agcd%3A75275456.

581. Open Science Foundation. Estimating the reproducibility of psychological science. Science. 2015;349(6251). Available from: http://science.sciencemag. org/sci/349/6251/aac4716.full.pdf.

582. Gøtzsche PC. Deadly psychiatry and organised denial: People'sPress; 2015.

583. Gøtzsche PC, Demasi M. Interventions to help patients withdraw from depression drugs: A systematic review. International Journal of Risk & Safety in Medicine. 2024;35:103-16. Available from: https://content.iospress. com/articles/international-journal-of-risk-and-safety-in-medicine/ jrs230011

https://www.medrxiv.org/content/10.1101/2023.03.13.23287182.full.pdf.

584. Davies J, GØtzsche PC, Timimi S, Moncrieff J, Montagu L, Breggin PR, et al. The sedated society

The Causes and Harms of our Psychiatric Drug Epidemic: Springer, Palgrave Macmillan; 2017. Available from: https://www.palgrave.com/gp/ media-centre/press/the-sedated-society/11994774.

585. Gøtzsche PC. Long-Term Use of Benzodiazepines, Stimulants and Lithium is Not Evidence-Based. Clin Neuropsychiatry. 2020;17(5):281-3. Available from: https://www.ncbi.nlm.nih.gov/pmc/articles/PMC8629043/.

586. Gøtzsche PC. Long-term use of antipsychotics and antidepressants is not evidence-based. International Journal of Risk & Safety in Medicine. 2020;31:37-42. Available from: https://content.iospress.com/articles/ international-journal-of-risk-and-safety-in-medicine/jrs195060

https://journals.sagepub.com/doi/full/10.3233/JRS-195060.

587. Gøtzsche PC. Critical psychiatry textbook2022. Available from: https:// www.scientificfreedom.dk/wp-content/uploads/2024/03/Gotzsche- Critical-Psychiatry-Textbook.pdf.

588. GØtzsche PC. Deadly Medicines & Organised Crime

A blog about drugs [Internet]2019. Available from: https://www. deadlymedicines.dk/the-harmful-myth-about-the-chemical-imbalance- causing-psychiatric-disorders/.

589. Taubes G, Mann CC. Epidemiology faces its limits. Science. 1995;269(5221):164- 9. Available from: https://www.science.org/doi/abs/10.1126/science.7618077

https://sethroberts.org/wp-content/uploads/2024/05/Taubes_limits_ epidemiology_Science_1995.pdf.

590. Montaner JSG, O'Shaughnessy MV, Schechter MT. Industry-sponsored clinical research: a double-edged sword. The Lancet. 2001;358(9296):1893- 5. Available from: http://www.sciencedirect.com/science/article/pii/ S014067360106891X.

591. Buchkowsky SS, Jewesson PJ. Industry Sponsorship and Authorship of Clinical Trials Over 20 Years. Annals of Pharmacotherapy. 2004;38(4):579-85. Available from: http://aop.sagepub.com/content/38/4/579.abstract.

592. Roseman M, Milette K, Bero LA, Coyne JC, Lexchin J, Turner EH, et al. Reporting of Conflicts of Interest in Meta-analyses of Trials of Pharmacological Treatments. JAMA. 2011;305(10):1008-17. Available from: https://doi.org/10.1001/jama.2011.257.

593. Carrick-Hagenbarth J, Epstein GA. Dangerous interconnectedness: economists' conflicts of interest, ideology and financial crisis. Cambridge Journal of Economics. 2012;36(1):43-63. Available from: https://doi.org/10.1093/cje/ber036.

594. Rose SL, Krzyzanowska MK, Joffe S. Relationships Between Authorship Contributions and Authors' Industry Financial Ties Among Oncology Clinical Trials. Journal of Clinical Oncology. 2010;28(8):1316-21. Available from: https://ascopubs.org/doi/abs/10.1200/JCO.2008.21.6606.

595. Tuckey TG, Hipwell RF. Plato's Charmides. 1953. Available from: https://www.cambridge.org/core/journals/journal-of-hellenic-studies/article/abs/platos-charmides-by-t-g-tuckey-pp-ix-116-cambridge-university-press-1951-12s-6d/84F706CF21392001E2E4C0A2BF18B778.

596. Code N. The Nuremberg Code, Declaration of Helsinki 1996 2000, Belmont Report. Trials of war criminals before the Nuremberg military tribunals under control council law. 1949(10):181-2. Available from: http://www.eddatatraining.net/assets/documents/ethics-references.pdf.

597. Schulz KF. Subverting randomization in controlled trials. JAMA. 1995;274 (18):1456-8. Available from: http://dx.doi.org/10.1001/jama.1995.03530180050029.

598. Gupta P, Gupta M, Koul N. Overdiagnosis and overtreatment; how to deal with too much medicine. Journal of Family Medicine and Primary Care. 2020;9(8):3815-9. Available from: https://journals.lww.com/jfmpc/fulltext/2020/09080/overdiagnosis_and_overtreatment__how_to_deal_with.5.aspx.

599. Frank E, Dresner Y, Shani M, Vinker S. The association between physicians' and patients' preventive health practices. Canadian Medical Association Journal. 2013:cmaj. 121028. Available from: https://www.cmaj.ca/content/185/8/649.short

https://www.cmaj.ca/content/cmaj/185/8/649.full.pdf.

600. McRae R. Salaried doctors: Healthy doctors fundamental for healthy patients. 2015. Available from: https://search.informit.org/doi/abs/10.3316/informit.033655276508040.

601. BMJ Editors. The BMJ 's wild goose chase. BMJ : British Medical Journal. 2002;325(7366):0-. Available from: http://www.ncbi.nlm.nih.gov/pmc/articles/PMC1124202/.

602. Davis DA, Thomson M, Oxman AD, Haynes R. Changing physician performance: A systematic review of the effect of continuing medical education strategies.

JAMA. 1995;274(9):700-5. Available from: http://dx.doi.org/10.1001/jama.1995.03530090032018.

603. Lindeman S, Läärä E, Hakko H, Lönnqvist J. A Systematic Review on Gender-Specific Suicide Mortality in Medical Doctors. British Journal of Psychiatry. 1996;168(3):274-9. Available from: https://www.cambridge.org/core/product/75ED952B056A57074B82A4BE6885E055.

604. Couto TCe, Rückl SCZ, Duarte D, Correa H. Suicide in Doctors. Suicide Risk Assessment and Prevention: Springer; 2022. p. 1-22. Available from: https://link.springer.com/content/pdf/10.1007/978-3-030-41319-4_29-1.pdf.

605. Ventriglio A, Watson C, Bhugra D. Suicide among doctors: A narrative review. Indian Journal of Psychiatry. 2020;62(2). Available from: https://journals.lww.com/indianjpsychiatry/fulltext/2020/62020/suicide_among_doctors__a_narrative_review.3.aspx.

606. Panagioti M, Geraghty K, Johnson J, Zhou A, Panagopoulou E, Chew-Graham C, et al. Association Between Physician Burnout and Patient Safety, Professionalism, and Patient Satisfaction: A Systematic Review and Meta-analysis. JAMA Intern Med. 2018;178(10):1317-31. Available from: https://www.ncbi.nlm.nih.gov/pubmed/30193239

https://jamanetwork.com/journals/jamainternalmedicine/articlepdf/2698144/jamainternal_panagioti_2018_oi_180055.pdf.

607. Maciosek MV, Coffield AB, Edwards NM, Flottemesch TJ, Goodman MJ, Solberg LI. Priorities Among Effective Clinical Preventive Services. American Journal of Preventive Medicine. 2006;31(1):52-61. Available from: http://dx.doi.org/10.1016/j.amepre.2006.03.012.

608. Cohen S. Nudging and informed consent. The American Journal of Bioethics. 2013;13(6):3-11. Available from: https://www.tandfonline.com/doi/abs/10.1080/15265161.2013.781704.

609. Hesse BW, Ahern DK, Woods SS. Nudging best practice: the HITECH act and behavioral medicine. Translational Behavioral Medicine. 2011;1(1):175-81. Available from: http://dx.doi.org/10.1007/s13142-010-0001-3.

610. Dai H, Saccardo S, Han MA, Roh L, Raja N, Vangala S, et al. Behavioural nudges increase COVID-19 vaccinations. Nature. 2021;597(7876):404-9. Available from: https://doi.org/10.1038/s41586-021-03843-2.

611. Tentori K, Pighin S, Giovanazzi G, Grignolio A, Timberlake B, Ferro A. Nudging COVID-19 Vaccine Uptake by Changing the Default: A Randomized Controlled Trial. Medical Decision Making. 2022;42(6):837-41. Available from: https://journals.sagepub.com/doi/abs/10.1177/0272989X221101536.

612. Reñosa MDC, Landicho J, Wachinger J, Dalglish SL, Bärnighausen K, Bärnighausen T, et al. Nudging toward vaccination: a systematic review. BMJ Global Health. 2021;6(9):e006237. Available from: https://gh.bmj.com/content/bmjgh/6/9/e006237.full.pdf.

613. Schenck D, Churchill L. Healers: extraordinary clinicians at work: Oxford University Press; 2011.

614. Churchill LR, Schenck D. Healing Skills for Medical Practice. Annals of Internal Medicine. 2008;149(10):720-4. Available from: https://www.acpjournals.org/doi/abs/10.7326/0003-4819-149-10-200811180-00006

615. Yates SW. Physician Stress and Burnout. The American Journal of Medicine. 2020;133(2):160-4. Available from: https://www.sciencedirect.com/science/article/pii/S0002934319307570.

616. Halbesleben JRB, Rathert C. Linking physician burnout and patient outcomes: Exploring the dyadic relationship between physicians and patients. Health Care Manage Rev. 2008;33(1):29-39. Available from: https://journals.lww.com/hcmrjournal/abstract/2008/01000/linking_physician_burnout_and_patient_outcomes_.5.aspx.

617. Dyrbye LN, Thomas MR, Shanafelt TD, editors. Medical student distress: causes, consequences, and proposed solutions. Mayo Clinic Proceedings; 2005: Elsevier. Available from: http://www.mayoclinicproceedings.org/article/S0025-6196(11)61057-4/pdf.

618. McManus I, Keeling A, Paice E. Stress, burnout and doctors' attitudes to work are determined by personality and learning style: a twelve year longitudinal study of UK medical graduates. BMC medicine. 2004;2(1):29. Available from: https://link.springer.com/article/10.1186/1741-7015-2-29.

619. Kay MP, Mitchell GK, Del Mar CBJMjoA. Doctors do not adequately look after their own physical health. Medical Journal of Australia. 2004;181(7):368. Available from: https://www.mja.com.au/system/files/issues/181_07_041004/kay10461_fm.pdf.

620. McDonald HP, Garg AX, Haynes RB. Interventions to enhance patient adherence to medication prescriptions: scientific review. Jama. 2002;288(22):2868-79. Available from: http://jama.jamanetwork.com/article.aspx?articleid=195605.

621. Dobson A, Byles J, Brown W, Mishra G, Loxton D, Hockey R, et al. Adherence to health guidelines: Findings from the Australian Longitudinal Study on Women's Health. 2012. Available from: https://alswh.org.au/wp-content/uploads/2022/03/2012_Major_Report_Adherence-to-health-guidelines.pdf.

622. Haynes R. Determinants of compliance. The disease and the mechanics of treatment. Baltimore MD, Johns Hopkins University Press; 1979.

623. Burke LE, Dunbar-Jacob JM, Hill MN. Compliance with cardiovascular disease prevention strategies: a review of the research. Annals of Behavioral Medicine. 1997;19(3):239-63. Available from: http://www.ncbi.nlm.nih.gov/pubmed/9603699.

624. Greenfield S, Kaplan S, Ware JE. Expanding patient involvement in care: effects on patient outcomes. Annals of internal medicine. 1985;102(4):520-8. Available from: http://annals.org/article.aspx?articleid=699554.

625. van Dulmen S, Sluijs E, van Dijk L, de Ridder D, Heerdink R, Bensing J. Patient adherence to medical treatment: a review of reviews. BMC health services research. 2007;7(1):55. Available from: http://www.biomedcentral.com/content/pdf/1472-6963-7-55.pdf.

626. Zolnierek KBH, DiMatteo MR. Physician communication and patient adherence to treatment: a meta-analysis. Med Care. 2009;47(8):826. Available from: http://www.ncbi.nlm.nih.gov/pmc/articles/PMC2728700/pdf/nihms109392.pdf.

627. Starfield B, Shi L. Policy relevant determinants of health: an international perspective. Health Policy. 2002;60(3):201-18. Available from: http://www.sciencedirect.com/science/article/pii/S0168851001002081.

628. Cooke M, Irby DM, Sullivan W, Ludmerer KM. American Medical Education 100 Years after the Flexner Report. New England Journal of Medicine. 2006;355(13):1339-44. Available from: http://www.nejm.org/doi/full/10.1056/NEJMra055445.

629. Landrigan CP, Rothschild JM, Cronin JW, Kaushal R, Burdick E, Katz JT, et al. Effect of reducing interns' work hours on serious medical errors in intensive care units. New England Journal of Medicine. 2004;351(18):1838-48. Available from: https://www.nejm.org/doi/full/10.1056/NEJMoa041406.

630. Barger LK, Cade BE, Ayas NT, Cronin JW, Rosner B, Speizer FE, et al. Extended Work Shifts and the Risk of Motor Vehicle Crashes among Interns. New England Journal of Medicine. 2005;352(2):125-34. Available from: http://www.nejm.org/doi/full/10.1056/NEJMoa041401.

631. Dimick JB. Association for Academic Surgery Presidential Address: The Rookie Advantage. Journal of Surgical Research. 2016. Available from: https://www.journalofsurgicalresearch.com/article/S0022-4804(16)00124-4/abstract.

632. Birkmeyer JD. Outcomes research and surgeons. Surgery. 1998;124(3):477-83. Available from: http://www.sciencedirect.com/science/article/pii/S0039606098700923.

633. Schmidt HG, van Gog T, CE Schuit S, Van den Berge K, LA Van Daele P, Bueving H, et al. Do patients' disruptive behaviours influence the accuracy of a doctor's diagnosis? A randomised experiment. BMJ Quality & Safety. 2016. Available from: http://qualitysafety.bmj.com/content/early/2016/02/09/bmjqs-2015-004109.abstract.

634. Kaplan SH, Greenfield S, Gandek B, Rogers WH, Ware JE. Characteristics of physicians with participatory decision-making styles. Annals of internal medicine. 1996;124(5):497-504. Available from: http://annals.org/article.aspx?articleid=709497

https://annals.org/aim/article-abstract/709497/characteristics-physicians-participatory-decision-making-styles.

635. Rowe L, Kidd M. Every Doctor

Healthier Doctors = Healthier Patients: CRC Press, Taylor & Francis Group; 2019.

636. Hurwitz B. What's a good doctor, and how can you make one? Bmj. 2002;325(7366):667-8. Available from: http://www.bmj.com/content/bmj/325/7366/667.full.pdf.

637. Rizo CA, Jadad AR, Enkin M. What's a good doctor and how do you make one? : Doctors should be good companions for people (BMJ Letters). BMJ :

British Medical Journal. 2002;325(7366):711-. Available from: http://www. ncbi.nlm.nih.gov/pmc/articles/PMC1124230/.

638. Blasi ZD, Harkness E, Ernst E, Georgiou A, Kleijnen J. Influence of context effects on health outcomes: a systematic review. The Lancet. 2001;357(9258):757-62. Available from: http://dx.doi.org/10.1016/S0140-6736(00)04169-6.

639. De Craen A, Kaptchuk TJ, Tijssen J, Kleijnen J. Placebos and placebo effects in medicine: historical overview. Journal of the Royal Society of Medicine. 1999;92(10):511. Available from: https://journals.sagepub.com/doi/abs/10.1177/014107689909201005.

640. Brody H. Placebos and the philosophy of medicine: Clinical, conceptual, and ethical issues. 1980.

641. Krogstad U, Hofoss D, Veenstra M, Hjortdahl P. Predictors of job satisfaction among doctors, nurses and auxiliaries in Norwegian hospitals: relevance for micro unit culture. Human Resources for Health. 2006;4(1):1-8. Available from: http://dx.doi.org/10.1186/1478-4491-4-3.

642. West E. Management matters: the link between hospital organisation and quality of patient care. Quality in Health Care. 2001;10(1):40-8. Available from: https://qualitysafety.bmj.com/content/10/1/40.short

https://pmc.ncbi.nlm.nih.gov/articles/PMC1743422/pdf/v010p00040.pdf.

643. Francis V, Korsch BM, Morris MJ. Gaps in Doctor-Patient Communication. New England Journal of Medicine. 1969;280(10):535-40. Available from: http://www.nejm.org/doi/full/10.1056/NEJM196903062801004.

644. Marinker M. From compliance to concordance: Royal Pharmaceutical Society, in partnership with Merck Sharp & Dohme, 1997; 1997. Available from: https://www.scirp.org/reference/referencespapers?reference id=286315.

645. Bissell P, May CR, Noyce PR. From compliance to concordance: barriers to accomplishing a re-framed model of health care interactions. Social Science & Medicine. 2004;58(4):851-62. Available from: http://www. sciencedirect.com/science/article/pii/S0277953603002594.

646. Vermeire E, Hearnshaw H, Van Royen P, Denekens J. Patient adherence to treatment: three decades of research. A comprehensive review. Journal of Clinical Pharmacy and Therapeutics. 2001;26(5):331-42. Available from: http://dx.doi.org/10.1046/j.1365-2710.2001.00363.x.

647. Bleich SN, Gudzune KA, Bennett WL, Jarlenski MP, Cooper LA. How does physician BMI impact patient trust and perceived stigma? Preventive medicine. 2013;57(2):120-4. Available from: http://www.ncbi.nlm.nih.gov/pmc/articles/PMC3745018/.

648. Puhl R, Gold J, Luedicke J, DePierre J. The effect of physicians' body weight on patient attitudes: implications for physician selection, trust and adherence to medical advice. International Journal of Obesity. 2013;37(11):1415-21. Available from: https://www.nature.com/articles/ijo201333

https://www.researchgate.net/profile/Rebecca-Puhl/publication/23
6060418_The_effect_of_physicians%27_body_weight_on_patient_attitudes_
Implications_for_physician_selection_trust_and_adherence_to_medical_
advice/links/547337df0cf24bc8ea19cf00/The-effect-of-physicians-body-
weight-on-patient-attitudes-Implications-for-physician-selection-trust-
and-adherence-to-medical-advice.pdf.

649. Frank E, Rothenberg R, Lewis C, Belodoff BF. Correlates of physicians'
prevention-related practices: findings from the Women Physicians'
Health Study. Archives of Family Medicine. 2000;9(4):359. Available from:
https://triggered.edina.clockss.org/ServeContent?url=http://archfami.
ama-assn.org%2Fcgi%2Fcontent%2Ffull%2F9%2F4%2F359.

650. Wells KB, Lewis CE, Leake B, Ware Jr JE. Do physicians preach what they
practice. JAMA. 1984;252:2846-8. Available from: https://jamanetwork.
com/journals/jama/article-abstract/395327.

651. Wright SM, Kern DE, Kolodner K, Howard DM, Brancati FL. Attributes
of excellent attending-physician role models. New England Journal of
Medicine. 1998;339(27):1986-93. Available from: http://www.nejm.org/
doi/full/10.1056/NEJM199812313392706.

652. Hattie J. The applicability of Visible Learning to higher education.
Scholarship of Teaching and Learning in Psychology. 2015;1(1):79-91.
Available from: https://psycnet.apa.org/buy/2015-13426-005.

653. Willett WC. Balancing Life-Style and Genomics Research for Disease
Prevention. Science. 2002;296(5568):695-8. Available from: http://www.
jstor.org/stable/3076576.

654. Tunstall-Pedoe H. Preventing Chronic Diseases. A Vital Investment: WHO
Global Report. Geneva: World Health Organization, 2005. pp 200. CHF 30.00.
ISBN 92 4 1563001. Also published on http://www.who.int/chp/chronic_
disease_report/en. International Journal of Epidemiology. 2006;35(4):1107.
Available from: http://ije.oxfordjournals.org/content/35/4/1107.short.

655. Kevin R. Campbell M. Heart health [Internet]. newsmax.com: newsmax
health. 2015. [cited 2016]. Available from: http://www.newsmax.com/
Health/KevinCampbell/kevin-campbell-doctor-heart/2015/05/06/
id/643021/

https://web.archive.org/web/*/http://www.newsmax.com/Health/
KevinCampbell/kevin-campbell-doctor-heart/2015/05/06/id/643021/.

656. Harrison S, Checkland K. Evidence-based practice in UK health policy. In:
Gabe J, Calnan M, editors. The new sociology of the health service. 1 ed.
Abigndon: Routledge; 2009. p. 121-42.

657. Regier DA, Kuhl EA, Kupfer DJ. The DSM-5: Classification and criteria
changes. World Psychiatry. 2013;12(2):92-8. Available from: https://
onlinelibrary.wiley.com/doi/abs/10.1002/wps.20050.

658. Boysen GA, Ebersole A. Expansion of the Concept of Mental Disorder in
the DSM-5. The Journal of Mind and Behavior. 2014;35(4):225-43. Available
from: http://www.jstor.org/stable/43854371.

659. Aylin P, Alexandrescu R, Jen MH, Mayer EK, Bottle A. Day of week of procedure and 30 day mortality for elective surgery: retrospective analysis of hospital episode statistics. BMJ. 2013;346. Available from: http://www.bmj.com/content/bmj/346/bmj.f2424.full.pdf

Video https://www.youtube.com/watch?v=eR7gwKBB6G0.

660. Imperial College London. Day of week of procedure and 30 day mortality for elective surgery. Youtube; 2013. Available from: https://www.youtube.com/watch?v=eR7gwKBB6G0.

661. Elizabeth Dolan JS, Joanne Brown, Matthew Brown, Sharon Gavioli, Narelle Kelly, Felicity Latchford, Francesca Leaton, Fiona Lotherington, Lee Poole, Kate Robson, Paula Steffensen Nurses General Submission to the Australian Parliament Senate Select Committee on Health. Senate Committee Submission. Australian Federal Parliament - Senate; 2014 22/10/2014. Contract No.: 107. Available from: http://www.aph.gov.au/Parliamentary_Business/Committees/Senate/Health/Health/Submissions.

662. Smith R. All doctors are problem doctors. Doctors worldwide must do better with managing problem colleagues. 1997;314(7084):841. Available from: https://www.bmj.com/content/314/7084/841.short

https://pmc.ncbi.nlm.nih.gov/articles/PMC2126232/pdf/9093086.pdf.

663. Lens P, van der Wal G. Problem doctors: a conspiracy of silence: IOS Press; 1997.

664. Trzeciak S, Gaughan JP, Bosire J, Mazzarelli AJ. Association Between Medicare Summary Star Ratings for Patient Experience and Clinical Outcomes in US Hospitals. Journal of Patient Experience. 2016;3(1):6-9. Available from: http://jpx.sagepub.com/content/3/1/6.abstract.

665. Drahota A, Ward D, Mackenzie H, Stores R, Higgins B, Gal D, et al. Sensory environment on health-related outcomes of hospital patients. Cochrane Database Syst Rev. 2012;3. Available from: http://dx.doi.org/10.1002/14651858.CD005315.pub2.

666. Ulrich R. View through a window may influence recovery. Science. 1984;224(4647):224-5. Available from: https://www.science.org/doi/abs/10.1126/science.6143402.

667. Ell K, Nishimoto R, Mediansky L, Mantell J, Hamovitch M. Social relations, social support and survival among patients with cancer. Journal of psychosomatic research. 1992;36(6):531-41. Available from: https://www.sciencedirect.com/science/article/abs/pii/0022399992900384.

668. Pearlman RA, Uhlmann RF. Quality of Life in Chronic Diseases: Perceptions of Elderly Patients. Journal of Gerontology. 1988;43(2):M25-M30. Available from: http://geronj.oxfordjournals.org/content/43/2/M25.abstract.

669. Weinberg NL, Robert. How Valeant Tripled Prices, Doubled Sales of Flatlining Drug: Bloomberg; 2016 [Available from: http://www.bloomberg.com/news/articles/2016-01-08/how-valeant-tripled-prices-doubled-sales-of-flatlining-old-drug.

670. Marshall B. Helicobacter connections - Noble lecture 2006. ChemMedChem. 2006;1(8):783-802. Available from: https://chemistry-europe.onlinelibrary. wiley.com/doi/abs/10.1002/cmdc.200600153

https://www.nobelprize.org/uploads/2018/06/marshall-lecture.pdf.

671. Marshall BW, Robin. ABC News Interview of 2005 Nobel Prize in Medicine Winners. 2005. Available from: http://www.rense.com/general67/discc. htm.

672. Tanenbaum J. Delayed Gratification: Why it Took Everybody So Long to Acknowledge that Bacteria Cause Ulcers. Journal of Young Investigators. 2005. Available from: http://www.jyi.org/issue/delayed-gratification-why-it-took-everybody-so-long-to-acknowledge-that-bacteria-cause-ulcers/.

673. Hill A, Simmons B, Gotham D, Fortunak J. Rapid reductions in prices for generic sofosbuvir and daclatasvir to treat hepatitis C. Journal of Virus Eradication. 2016;2:28-31. Available from: https://www.sciencedirect. com/science/article/pii/S2055664020306919

674. Shepard CW, Finelli L, Alter MJ. Global epidemiology of hepatitis C virus infection. The Lancet Infectious Diseases. 2005;5(9):558-67. Available from: http://dx.doi.org/10.1016/S1473-3099(05)70216-4.

675. Jansen NA. Clarifications Needed on Study of Association between Physician Burnout and Patient Safety. JAMA Internal Medicine. 2019;179(4):592-3. Available from: https://jamanetwork.com/journals/jamainternal medicine/article-abstract/2726047.

676. Panagioti M, Hodkinson A, Esmail A. Clarifications Needed on Study of Association between Physician Burnout and Patient Safety - Reply. JAMA Internal Medicine. 2019;179(4):593-4. Available from: https://jamanetwork. com/journals/jamainternalmedicine/article-abstract/2726049.

677. Dyrbye LN, Shanafelt TD, West CP. Clarifications Needed on Study of Association between Physician Burnout and Patient Safety. JAMA Internal Medicine. 2019;179(4):592-3. Available from: https://jamanetwork.com/ journals/jamainternalmedicine/article-abstract/2726047.

678. Brown ME, Treviño LK. Do Role Models Matter? An Investigation of Role Modeling as an Antecedent of Perceived Ethical Leadership. Journal of Business Ethics. 2014;122(4):587-98. Available from: http://dx.doi. org/10.1007/s10551-013-1769-0.

679. Cruess SR, Cruess RL, Steinert Y. Teaching Rounds: Role Modelling: Making the Most of a Powerful Teaching Strategy. BMJ: British Medical Journal. 2008;336(7646):718-21. Available from: http://www.jstor.org/ stable/20509341.

680. Paice E, Heard S, Moss F. How important are role models in making good doctors? Br Med J. 2002;325(7366):707.

681. Jochemsen-van der Leeuw HGAR, van Dijk N, van Etten-Jamaludin FS, Wieringa-de Waard M. The Attributes of the Clinical Trainer as a Role Model: A Systematic Review. Academic Medicine. 2013;88(1):26-34. Available

from: http://journals.lww.com/academicmedicine/Fulltext/2013/01000/ The_Attributes_of_the_Clinical_Trainer_as_a_Role.16.aspx.

682. Wright S, Wong A, Newill C. The Impact of Role Models on Medical Students. J Gen Intern Med. 1997;12(1):53-6. Available from: http://dx.doi. org/10.1046/j.1525-1497.1997.12109.x.

683. Morgan M. The doctor-patient relationship. Sociology as applied to medicine. 2003:49-65.

684. Wang YC, McPherson K, Marsh T, Gortmaker SL, Brown M. Health and economic burden of the projected obesity trends in the USA and the UK. The Lancet. 2011;378(9793):815-25. Available from: https://www.thelancet. com/journals/lancet/article/PIIS0140-6736(11)60814-3/abstract

https://www.sochob.cl/pdf/obesidad_adulto/Obesity%202%20Health%20 and%20economic%20burden%20of%20the%20projected%20obesity%20 trends.pdf.

685. Aljadani H, Sibbritt D, Patterson A, Collins C. The Australian Recommended Food Score did not predict weight gain in middle-aged Australian women during six years of follow-up. Australian and New Zealand journal of public health. 2013;37(4):322-8. Available from: https://www.sciencedirect.com/ science/article/pii/S1326020023008671.

686. De Cocker KA, Van Uffelen JG, Brown WJ. Associations between sitting time and weight in young adult Australian women. Preventive medicine. 2010;51(5):361-7. Available from: https://www.sciencedirect.com/science/ article/abs/pii/S0091743510002884.

687. Raatikainen P. Gödel's Incompleteness Theorems. The Stanford Encyclopedia of Philosophy [Internet]. 2015. Available from: http://plato.stanford.edu/ entries/goedel-incompleteness/.

688. Schnelle C. What makes an exceptionally good doctor? [PhD by Publication]. Robina, Australia: Bond University; 2023. Available from: https://research. bond.edu.au/en/studentTheses/what-makes-an-exceptionally-good- doctor.

689. Bauval R, Hancock G. Keeper of Genesis: A Quest for the Hidden Legacy of Mankind. London: Mandarin Paperbacks; 1997.

690. Kübler-Ross E. On death and dying: What the dying have to teach doctors, nurses, clergy and their own families

40th anniversary edition: Taylor & Francis; 2009.

691. Becker E. The denial of death: Simon and Schuster; 2007.

692. Shah SK, Miller FG. Can we handle the truth? Legal fictions in the determination of death. American journal of law & medicine. 2010;36(4):540- 85. Available from: https://www.cambridge.org/core/journals/ american-journal-of-law-and-medicine/article/abs/can-we-handle-the- truth-legal-fictions-in-the-determination-of-death/265EF02A0E3C6B06 AB5B8203C83280DE.

693. Willett WC. Diet and health: what should we eat? Science. 1994;264(5158):532- 7. Available from: https://www.science.org/doi/abs/10.1126/science.8160011.

694. Breslow L. Behavioral factors in the health status of urban populations. Journal of Urban Health : Bulletin of the New York Academy of Medicine. 1998;75(2):242-50. Available from: http://www.ncbi.nlm.nih.gov/pmc/articles/PMC3456245/.

695. Breslow L, Breslow N. Health practices and disability: some evidence from Alameda County. Preventive Medicine. 1993;22(1):86-95. Available from: https://www.sciencedirect.com/science/article/abs/pii/S0091743583710066.

696. Brown JS, McCreedy M. The hale elderly: Health behavior and its correlates. Research in Nursing & Health. 1986;9(4):317-29. Available from: http://dx.doi.org/10.1002/nur.4770090409

https://onlinelibrary.wiley.com/doi/10.1002/nur.4770090409.

697. Lee PI, Hu YL, Chen PY, Huang YC, Hsueh PR. Are children less susceptible to COVID-19? J Microbiol Immunol Infect. 2020;53(3):371-2. Available from: https://pmc.ncbi.nlm.nih.gov/articles/PMC7102573/

https://www.sciencedirect.com/science/article/pii/S1684118220300396.

698. Kostoff RN, Calina D, Kanduc D, Briggs MB, Vlachoyiannopoulos P, Svistunov AA, et al. RETRACTED: Why are we vaccinating children against COVID-19? Toxicology Reports. 2021;8:1665-84. Available from: https://www.sciencedirect.com/science/article/pii/S221475002100161X.

699. Halma MTJ, Rose J, Lawrie T. The Novelty of mRNA Viral Vaccines and Potential Harms: A Scoping Review. J. 2023;6(2):220-35. Available from: https://www.mdpi.com/2571-8800/6/2/17.

700. Bitounis D, Jacquinet E, Rogers MA, Amiji MM. Strategies to reduce the risks of mRNA drug and vaccine toxicity. Nature Reviews Drug Discovery. 2024;23(4):281-300. Available from: https://doi.org/10.1038/s41573-023-00859-3.

701. Chavda VP, Jogi G, Dave S, Patel BM, Vineela Nalla L, Koradia K. mRNA-Based Vaccine for COVID-19: They Are New but Not Unknown! Vaccines. 2023;11(3):507. Available from: https://www.mdpi.com/2076-393X/11/3/507.

INDEX

Printed in Great Britain
by Amazon

57680590R00228